# Clinical
# Prediction
# Rules

MW00340435

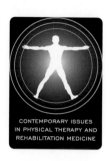

Jones and Bartlett's
*Contemporary Issues in Physical Therapy and Rehabilitation Medicine* Series

## Series Editor

Peter A. Huijbregts, PT, MSc, MHSc, DPT, OCS, FAAOMPT, FCAMT

## Books in the Series

### Now Available

*Tension-Type and Cervicogenic Headache:*
*Pathophysiology, Diagnosis, and Management*
César Fernández-de-las-Peñas, PT, DO, PhD
Lars Arendt-Nielsen, DMSc, PhD
Robert D. Gerwin, MD

*Myofascial Trigger Points:*
*Pathophysiology and Evidence-Informed Diagnosis and Management*
Jan Dommerholt, PT, DPT, MPS, DAAPM
Peter A. Huijbregts, PT, MSc, MHSc, DPT, OCS, FAAOMPT, FCAMT

*Wellness and Physical Therapy*
Sharon Elayne Fair, PT, MS, PhD

*Orthopaedic Manual Therapy Diagnosis: Spine and Temporomandibular Joints*
Aad van der El, BPE, BSc, PT, Dip. MT, Dip. Acupuncture

### Coming Soon

*Post-Surgical Rehabilitation After Artificial Disc Replacement:*
*An Evidenced-Based Guide to Comprehensive Patient Care*
John N. Flood, DO, FACOS, FAOAO
Roy Bechtel, PT, PhD
Scott Benjamin, PT, DScPT

# Clinical Prediction Rules

## A Physical Therapy Reference Manual

Paul E. Glynn, PT, DPT, OCS, FAAOMPT
Supervisor of Staff Development and Clinical Research
Rehabilitation Department
Newton-Wellesley Hospital
Newton, Massachusetts

P. Cody Weisbach, PT, DPT
Physical Therapist
Rehabilitation Department
Newton-Wellesley Hospital
Newton, Massachusetts

UNIVERSITY OF SASKATCHEWAN

LIBRARY

**JONES AND BARTLETT PUBLISHERS**

*Sudbury, Massachusetts*

BOSTON    TORONTO    LONDON    SINGAPORE

Health Sciences Library
University of Saskatchewan Libraries
Room B205 Health Sciences Building
107 WIGGINS ROAD
SASKATOON, SK  S7N 5E5  CANADA

MAR 09 2010

*World Headquarters*

Jones and Bartlett Publishers
40 Tall Pine Drive
Sudbury, MA 01776
978-443-5000
info@jbpub.com
www.jbpub.com

Jones and Bartlett Publishers Canada
6339 Ormindale Way
Mississauga, Ontario L5V 1J2
Canada

Jones and Bartlett Publishers International
Barb House, Barb Mews
London W6 7PA
United Kingdom

Jones and Bartlett's books and products are available through most bookstores and online booksellers. To contact Jones and Bartlett Publishers directly, call 800-832-0034, fax 978-443-8000, or visit our website, www.jbpub.com.

Substantial discounts on bulk quantities of Jones and Bartlett's publications are available to corporations, professional associations, and other qualified organizations. For details and specific discount information, contact the special sales department at Jones and Bartlett via the above contact information or send an email to specialsales@jbpub.com.

Copyright © 2011 by Jones and Bartlett Publishers, LLC

All rights reserved. No part of the material protected by this copyright may be reproduced or utilized in any form, electronic or mechanical, including photocopying, recording, or by any information storage and retrieval system, without written permission from the copyright owner.

The authors, editor, and publisher have made every effort to provide accurate information. However, they are not responsible for errors, omissions, or for any outcomes related to the use of the contents of this book and take no responsibility for the use of the products and procedures described. Treatments and side effects described in this book may not be applicable to all people; likewise, some people may require a dose or experience a side effect that is not described herein. Drugs and medical devices are discussed that may have limited availability controlled by the Food and Drug Administration (FDA) for use only in a research study or clinical trial. Research, clinical practice, and government regulations often change the accepted standard in this field. When consideration is being given to use of any drug in the clinical setting, the health care provider or reader is responsible for determining FDA status of the drug, reading the package insert, and reviewing prescribing information for the most up-to-date recommendations on dose, precautions, and contraindications, and determining the appropriate usage for the product. This is especially important in the case of drugs that are new or seldom used.

**Production Credits**

Chief Executive Officer: Clayton Jones
Chief Operating Officer: Don W. Jones, Jr.
President, Higher Education and Professional Publishing: Robert W. Holland, Jr.
V.P., Sales: William J. Kane
V.P., Design and Production: Anne Spencer
V.P., Manufacturing and Inventory Control: Therese Connell
Publisher: David Cella
Associate Editor: Maro Gartside
Production Manager: Julie Champagne Bolduc

Production Assistant: Jessica Steele Newfell
Marketing Manager: Grace Richards
Manufacturing and Inventory Control Supervisor: Amy Bacus
Interior Design and Composition: Shawn Girsberger
Cover and Title Page Design: Kristin E. Parker
Cover Image: © Gary Cookson/ShutterStock, Inc.
Printing and Binding: Replika Press
Cover Printing: Replika Press

**Library of Congress Cataloging-in-Publication Data**
Glynn, Paul E.
  Clinical prediction rules : a physical therapy reference manual / Paul E. Glynn, P. Cody Weisbach.
     p. ; cm.
  Includes bibliographical references and index.
  ISBN 978-0-7637-7518-6 (pbk. : alk. paper)
  1. Physical therapy—Handbooks, manuals, etc. 2. Medical protocols—Handbooks, manuals, etc. I. Weisbach, P. Cody (Philip Cody) II. Title.
  [DNLM: 1. Musculoskeletal Diseases—rehabilitation—Adult—Handbooks. 2. Decision Support Techniques—Adult—Handbooks. 3. Physical Therapy Modalities—Adult—Handbooks. WE 39 G568c 2010]
  RM701.G57 2010
  615.8'2—dc22
                                                                                          2009031528

6048
Printed in India
13 12 11 10 09   10 9 8 7 6 5 4 3 2 1

*To my wife, Buquet, and my daughter, Emma—*
*thank you for your love, support, and patience.*
*You mean the world to me.*
*PG*

*For Cara . . . my favorite.*
*CW*

# BRIEF CONTENTS

# CONTENTS

## 6   Upper Extremities                                                 119

# FOREWORD

*Clinical Prediction Rules: A Physical Therapy Reference Manual* by Drs. Paul Glynn and P. Cody Weisbach will make a substantial and timely contribution to the physical therapy profession. The profession recently experienced an influx in the development of clinical prediction rules (CPRs), which provide physical therapists with an evidence-based tool to assist in patient management when determining a particular diagnosis or prognosis, or when predicting a response to a particular intervention. Clinicians often are left without evidence to guide clinical decision making. CPRs make terrific contributions to the evidence available to physical therapists and will greatly enhance the quality of care provided to patients. Drs. Glynn and Weisbach have taken the first step in the much-needed process of ensuring that CPRs are used on a consistent basis. They have provided a user-friendly guide to understanding the principles and utilization of CPRs in physical therapy practice. Furthermore, *Clinical Prediction Rules: A Physical Therapy Reference Manual* provides an extensive list of CPRs that have been developed and the potential implications for the patients whom physical therapists treat.

Despite the increasing popularity of CPRs, they are not without limitations and should be subjected to the scientific scrutiny of continued methodologically sound research. The authors of this text have clearly identified that CPRs in the initial stage of development should be used with caution and only within the context of the existing risks and benefits. Evidence provided through the use of uncontrolled cohort studies—which often are used in the development of CPRs—should not be defended as an endpoint but rather as the first step in the research process. Despite the fact that the majority of CPRs useful to physical therapists exist in the initial stages of development, in the absence of strong evidence, they are capable of providing useful information to the clinician that may in turn enhance patient outcomes. The authors have provided readers with all of the tools necessary to decide whether a CPR is appropriate for the patient sitting before them. Furthermore, this text lucidly identifies common methodological flaws associated with CPR studies and provides a quality assessment score for all derivation-level studies of which an assessment tool exists. This will greatly enhance the ability of physical therapists to critique CPRs and determine their applicability to clinical practice. Drs. Glynn and Weisbach emphasize the need to determine a rule's accuracy in different practice settings and its impact on outcomes of care and costs. The caveat is that clinicians cannot be entirely confident in the accuracy of a rule's use until more definitive validation studies are completed. For this reason, the authors did not include CPRs that have not been validated if the magnitude of the decision being made is such that the risk of making an inaccurate decision exceeds the potential benefits (e.g., the potential of a false negative for cervical spine fracture).

Clinical prediction rules should not be construed as removal of the clinical decision-making process from physical therapist practice. Instead, they should be used to eliminate some of the uncertainty that occurs with each and every clinical encounter and to provide a level of evidence on which clinicians can make decisions with adequate confidence. Sticking with the principles of evidence-based practice, the authors encourage therapists to incorporate the best available evidence (including CPRs) combined with clinical expertise and patient values to enhance the overall quality of care provided to individual patients.

I am certain we will continue to see the use of CPRs assist in advancing clinical practice in the physical therapy profession. Because it will be increasingly difficult for busy clinicians to stay abreast of the current best evidence, this text will assist in alleviating the complicated process of synthesizing the evidence. *Clinical Prediction Rules: A Physical Therapy Reference Manual* provides a succinct and clear guide to the use of CPRs in clinical practice and will prove an invaluable tool for both students and physical therapists in maximizing the quality of care provided to patients. This text is much more than a compendium of CPRs, and it will serve to improve the understanding of the clinical implications of CPRs and should enhance the translation of evidence to clinical practice. The authors should be congratulated, as the text clearly achieves its goal of serving as a clinical resource and reference manual to a collection of clinical prediction rules pertinent to the outpatient, orthopaedic physical therapist.

*Joshua A. Cleland, PT, PhD*
*Professor*
*Franklin Pierce University*
*Concord, New Hampshire*

# ACKNOWLEDGMENTS

Without the help of many, this book would not be possible. For this reason, we would like to acknowledge the following:

- Jones and Bartlett Publishers for its attention to detail and dedication to this endeavor.
- Tim Flynn, PT, PhD, OCS, FAAOMPT, Regis University, Denver, Colorado; Chad Cook, PT, PhD, MBA, OCS, COMT, Duke University, Durham, North Carolina; Gary Austin, PT, PhD, OCS, Sacred Heart University, Fairfield, Connecticut; Bill Egan, PT, DPT, OCS, FAAOMPT, Temple University, Philadelphia, Pennsylvania; and César Fernández-de-las-Peñas, PT, DO, PhD, Universidad Rey Juan Carlos, Madrid, Spain, for their review of our manuscript and their thoughtful suggestions to help improve its quality.
- Amber Hosey, PT, DPT, for her consistent clinical feedback as well as for agreeing to model for the photos in this text.
- The Rehabilitation Department of Newton-Wellesley Hospital for its commitment to quality patient care, evidence-based practice, and the education of future physical therapists.

To all, we thank you!

I think it is safe to say that the advent of clinical prediction rules has caused quite a stir in the orthopaedic physical therapy world. Clinical prediction rules are decision-making tools that contain predictor variables obtained from patient history, examination, and simple diagnostic tests; they can assist in making a diagnosis, establishing a prognosis, or determining appropriate management strategies.[1] In other words, clinical prediction rules (CPRs) are diagnostic, prognostic, or interventional/prescriptive. To date, the large majority of clinical prediction rules within the physical therapy literature are prescriptive in nature. Prescriptive clinical prediction rules are an exponent of the treatment-based system. In this type of diagnostic classification system, a cluster of signs and symptoms from the patient history and physical examination is used to classify patients into subgroups with specific implications for management.[2] As such, it produces homogeneous subgroups where all subjects within that group are expected to respond favorably to a matched intervention. All orthopaedic physical therapists will be able to recall various systematic reviews and meta-analyses published in leading biomedical journals that have indicated interventions that we know to be effective in our everyday clinical practice. These reviews are either no more effective than the standard of care or have an effect size similar to placebo interventions. A 2003 meta-analysis showing a lack of evidence for the use of manipulation in the management of patients with low back pain can serve as an often-referenced illustration.[3] Not that this finding should surprise us: If studies included in a systematic review or meta-analysis use no patient classification other than a broad category of nonspecific regional pain, the resultant heterogeneous study samples pretty much preclude finding real effects of even the most effective intervention.[4] Their ability to identify homogeneous subgroups immediately makes the development and validation of prescriptive clinical prediction rules a priority for our profession. As *Clinical Prediction Rules: A Physical Therapy Reference Manual* shows, many researchers have indeed recognized this importance, and the result is the impressive number of clinical prediction rules presented in this text.

So why has the development and application of clinical prediction rules, particularly prescriptive rules, led to such controversy in orthopaedic physical therapy? One obvious reason is the fear that such rules may lead to a loss of autonomy with regard to clinical decision making. In this context, the choice of the word *prescriptive* has been less than fortuitous. And, admittedly, this fear is grounded in reality. Colleagues have told me that some healthcare organizations instituted company-wide educational programs and policies that (inappropriately and prematurely) positioned the application of nonvalidated clinical prediction rules as the new standard of care. As with any research, there is the potential that interested third parties use their findings to inappropriately limit care and reimbursement. Another reason for this fear is that clinical prediction rules may seem hard to integrate with the mechanism-based classification system still used as the predominant paradigm by many orthopaedic physical therapists today. This paradigm is based on the premise that impairments identified during examination are the cause of musculoskeletal pain and dysfunction; interventions aimed at resolving these impairments are assumed to lead to decreased pain and increased function.[5]

Why is—despite these concerns—this book a worthwhile text that should ideally be included in the professional library of all orthopaedic physical therapists as well as of other conservative musculoskeletal care providers? First, clinical prediction rules were never intended to replace mechanism-based decision making. As with all research, we need to take into account external validity, which means that we can only apply clinical prediction rule research to patient populations that are sufficiently similar to the populations in which the tool was developed or validated. Acknowledging that the majority of clinical decisions will still be made using the mechanism-based paradigm, clinical prediction rules simply provide us with another tool for a specific subpopulation, albeit that for this subpopulation it provides a higher level of support from research evidence than does reasoning using the mechanism-based paradigm. However, to appropriately use this extra tool in our clinical toolbox, we need to know about content and relevance to our clinical practice of the clinical prediction rule. Second, any clinician will want to guard against misinterpretation and misuse of this tool for the purpose of limiting therapist autonomy and patient care. This means we need to be aware of limitations not only relevant to the individual rules but also inherent in the research process involved in deriving and validating these rules.

*Clinical Prediction Rules: A Physical Therapy Reference Manual* provides ready access to the clinical prediction rules relevant to orthopaedic clinical practice. It starts with a discussion of rules used for screening patients for the need for referral, followed by a presentation of rules organized by body region, and further divided into diagnostic, prognostic, and interventional rules. Taking into account the dire consequences of incorrect decisions during the screening portion of the examination, only screening rules that have undergone broad-based validation are included. An in-depth but accessible discussion of the research process, common methodological shortcomings in clinical prediction rule research, and relevant statistics provide the clinician with the tools required for critical analysis and appropriate application. Methodological quality scores are provided for prognostic and prescriptive rules and for validation studies. In the absence of a validated methodological quality assessment tool for diagnostic studies, the authors have proposed and provided a quality checklist for such studies. This allows for further critical interpretation by the clinician interested in application of the rules in clinical practice. Current, evidence-informed, and patient-centered clinical practice in orthopaedic physical therapy and other conservative musculoskeletal care professions requires the clinician to provide care based on an integration of current best research evidence, clinician expertise, and patient preferences. This text provides not only the current best evidence but also adds to clinician expertise by providing the tools required for critical analysis of this evidence. Finally, by providing the clinician with the knowledge required to educate the patient with regard to appropriate interpretation of clinical prediction rules, it also allows for truly informed patient input in the clinical decision-making process.

*Peter A. Huijbregts, PT, MSc, MHSc, DPT, OCS, FAAOMPT, FCAMT*
*Series Editor,* Contemporary Issues in Physical Therapy and Rehabilitation
  Medicine
*Victoria, British Columbia, Canada*

## References

1. Laupacis A, Sekar N, Stiell I. Clinical prediction rules: a review and suggested modification of methodological standards. *JAMA*. 1997;277:488–494.
2. Delitto A, Erhard RE, Bowling RW. A treatment-based classification approach to low back syndrome: identifying and staging patients for conservative treatment. *Phys Ther*. 1995;75:470–485.
3. Assendelft WJJ, Morton SC, Yu EI, Suttorp MJ, Shekelle PG. Spinal manipulative therapy for low back pain: a meta-analysis of effectiveness relative to other therapies. *Ann Intern Med*. 2003;138:871–881.
4. Childs JD, Flynn TW. Spinal manipulation for low back pain. *Ann Intern Med*. 2004;140:665.
5. Van Dillen LR, Sahrmann SA, Norton BJ, et al. Reliability of physical examination items used for classification of patients with low back pain. *Phys Ther*. 1998;78:979–988.

## Paul E. Glynn, PT, DPT, OCS, FAAOMPT

Dr. Glynn graduated from the University of Massachusetts at Lowell with a BS in Exercise Physiology and later earned his MS in Physical Therapy in 1997. In 2001, he completed a Certificate of Advanced Studies in Orthopaedic Physical Therapy as well as his Doctorate in Physical Therapy from the MGH Institute of Health Professions in Boston, Massachusetts. Dr. Glynn achieved board certification as an Orthopaedic Clinical Specialist in 2002. In 2006, he completed his manual therapy fellowship training at Regis University in Denver, Colorado, and he currently serves as affiliate faculty in the university's transitional DPT and fellowship programs. Dr. Glynn also serves as affiliate faculty at the University of Medicine and Dentistry in Newark, New Jersey, as well as for Evidence in Motion, Inc. in Louisville, Kentucky. Currently he works as the Supervisor of Staff Development and Clinical Research at Newton-Wellesley Hospital in Newton, Massachusetts, where he is a member of the Institutional Review Board.

Dr. Glynn has published research in numerous peer-reviewed journals, including *Physical Therapy*, the *Journal of Manual and Manipulative Therapy*, the *Journal of Sports Rehabilitation*, and the *Journal of Shoulder and Elbow Surgery*. He is the recipient of the 2006 Excellence in Research Award, the JMMT Therapeutic Exercise Award, and the 2008 Jack Walker Award. He is an active researcher and national presenter in the field, a manuscript reviewer for the *Journal of Manual and Manipulative Therapy*, and an item writer for the National Physical Therapy Exam (NPTE) and the Specialization Academy of Content Experts (SACE). Dr. Glynn also is an associate member of the Federation of State Boards of Physical Therapy (FSBPT) and has recently served on the FSBPT's standards setting task force for the NPTE.

## P. Cody Weisbach, PT, DPT

Dr. Weisbach earned his BA in Kinesiology and Applied Physiology from the University of Colorado at Boulder and completed his Doctorate in Physical Therapy at Simmons College in Boston, Massachusetts, in 2007. He is currently enrolled in a manual therapy fellowship at Regis University in Denver, Colorado.

Since graduation, Dr. Weisbach has worked with an orthopaedic population in a hospital-based outpatient setting at Newton-Wellesley Hospital in Newton, Massachusetts. In addition to his clinical duties, he has acted as a clinical investigator for several studies pending publication and is the primary investigator of a study investigating the effects of manual physical therapy applied to the hip in patients with low back pain. Dr. Weisbach has been published in *Physical Therapy* and recently participated in a clinical commentary on the influence of the hip in lower-back pain published in the *Journal of Sports Rehabilitation*.

Dr. Weisbach has been active in the American Physical Therapy Association (APTA) since 2004 and is a member of the Orthopaedic Section of the APTA and the American Academy of Orthopaedic Manual Physical Therapists.

# INTRODUCTION

The field of physical therapy (PT) has been undergoing a paradigm shift recently as the importance of evidence in practice is realized. Evidence-based medicine has been defined as the conscientious, explicit, and judicious use of the best available evidence.[1] Effective use of the current evidence requires the clinician to draw on clinical experience and assess patient values as well as to collect, analyze, and implement the available high-quality research. The process of incorporating evidence into physical therapy practice can be quite challenging as the literature continues to grow and evolve at a seemingly insurmountable pace. To further complicate decision making, the interventions used in high-quality research are often controlled to such an extent that their results may not be realistically applied to individual patients in everyday practice. Given these challenges, the physical therapist would benefit from tools specifically aimed at facilitating evidence-based diagnostic, prognostic, and interventional decision making. One such tool has existed for decades within the medical literature but has only recently begun to appear in the PT research; it is called the clinical prediction rule.

## Definition

Clinical prediction rules (CPRs) are algorithmic decision tools designed to aid clinicians in determining a diagnosis, prognosis, or likely response to an intervention. They use a parsimonious set of clinical findings from the history, physical examination, and diagnostic test results that have been analyzed and found to be statistically meaningful predictors of a condition or outcome of interest.[2–10] One example is a CPR by Flynn et al.[11] to identify patients with acute low back pain (LBP) who will benefit from lumbar manipulation. The authors found five variables that were associated with success from manipulation: duration of symptoms less than 16 days, symptoms do not extend below the knee, hypomobility in at least one lumbar spine segment, either hip with internal rotation greater than 35°, and a Fear–Avoidance Beliefs Questionnaire Work subscale score of less than 19. The authors found that patients who possess four or more of the above variables are likely to benefit from lumbar manipulation.

CPRs use statistical models to identify the complex interaction of predictive variables in clinical practice. They are in turn able to help guide the clinician and provide him or her with a more efficient way to accurately subgroup patients while also reducing potential biases.[4–6,9] CPRs are therefore highly useful in situations where decision making is complex due to heterogeneous conditions (e.g., LBP), the clinical stakes are high (e.g., deep vein thrombosis), or there is an opportunity for cost savings without compromising the quality of care (e.g., ordering of radiographs).[7,12]

There are three distinct types of CPRs: diagnostic, prognostic, and interventional. Diagnostic CPRs (DCPRs) help clinicians determine the probability that a patient has a particular condition. Prognostic CPRs (PCPRs) provide information about the likely outcome of patients with a specific condition, and interventional CPRs (ICPRs), also called prescriptive CPRs, aid clinicians in determining which patients are likely to respond favorably to an intervention or set of interventions.[2–10]

# CPR Development

Before initiating the development of a CPR the need for such a tool should be identified. The greatest need is believed to be in highly prevalent conditions characterized by diagnostic uncertainty, diagnostic heterogeneity, or high practice variability.[12–14] The process of preplanning for CPR development aids the researcher in identifying areas where an evidence base for clinical decision making is lacking, thus potentially improving the clinical utility of the tool.

CPRs exist along a continuum of quality and validity for clinical use. According to McGinn et al,[7] progress along this continuum involves a three-step process: derivation, validation, and impact analysis. CPRs can also be graded on a scale from I to IV depending on where they are on the developmental continuum with Level I indicating the highest stage of development and Level IV indicating the lowest. Those that have been derived but have yet to undergo validation or impact analysis are considered Level IV.[3,4,7,9] The progression from a Level IV to a Level III CPR includes validation of the original variable set in a "narrow" population (i.e., similar to the derivation study). This often involves examining the predictive value of the CPR in a separate population within the original derivation study. Due to the similar nature of the two samples, these CPRs still demonstrate limited generalizability into PT practice. CPRs that have been validated in "broad" populations (i.e., larger, more diverse patient samples) are considered Level II prediction rules. These rules can be applied confidently in clinical care as they have demonstrated stability in their predictive ability across diverse populations. Lastly, CPRs that have been implemented on a large scale and have demonstrated the ability to affect the quality and/or economy of care are considered Level I.[3,4,7,9] To help the clinician better understand the development process a brief description of each step is included.

## Derivation

Although many research designs may be utilized to derive a CPR (e.g., randomized clinical trials, retrospective analyses, cross-sectional analyses), currently the prospective cohort design is most frequently used in the PT literature.[9] In such a design, a group of patients are selected based upon specific inclusion and exclusion criteria. All patients undergo a standardized examination, receive a reference standard test (DCPRs), specific treatment (ICPRs), or wait a specified period of time (PCPRs) and finally undergo an outcomes assessment. With this study design there is no comparison or control group.[9]

The derivation process begins by selecting the target condition through the preplanning process described earlier (e.g., conditions lacking evidence, treatment variability).[4,7,9] Once the target condition has been chosen, the outcome of interest must be clearly defined so the clinician may accurately frame his or her expected outcome and the most appropriate measures can be selected.[3–10] For DCPRs this means using the most reliable and valid reference standard available to ensure that the condition is properly identified. In the case of ICPRs and PCPRs, it is important to use outcome measures with strong psychometric properties. The outcome tools should possess a recognized acceptable level of measurement error to help confirm statistically meaningful change; this is known as the minimal detectable change (MDC).[15] They should also possess a difference score determined to be clinically meaningful to the patient, which is referred to as the minimal clinically important difference or (MCID).[16] The use of such statistically sound measures helps to improve the likelihood that recorded changes are significant, meaningful, and are not due to chance.

Once the reference standard and/or outcome measures have been selected, the set of potential predictor variables must be established. These are all of the items that will be examined during the study for their relationship to the desired outcome. Potential predictor variables may include items from the history, physical exam, and self-report instruments (including psychosocial factors). The researchers must find a balance between choosing a select list of potential predictor variables, since the data will likely be collected under the time constraints typical of a busy clinical setting, while still including all relevant variables that might improve the predictive ability of the CPR.[5,7,9] For this reason reliable and valid variables are often identified through prior research studies. However, if such research is lacking, a larger set of predictor variables may be chosen based upon clinical experience and expert opinion. This comprehensive approach helps to minimize the likelihood that a potential predictor variable is overlooked.

After undergoing a standardized historical and physical examination, the patients receive either the reference standard test (DCPRs), the treatment under investigation (ICPRs), or they wait a predetermined amount of time (PCPRs). The outcome(s) for each subject is (are) then determined. In most CPRs the outcome is dichotomized into two distinct possibilities. For DCPRs, the reference standard test is used to determine the presence or absence of the target condition. In the case of both ICPRs and PCPRs the outcome measure is used to determine whether the patient is either "successful" or "nonsuccessful" or whether symptoms are persistent or nonpersistent.

To determine successful from nonsuccessful, the investigators will establish the magnitude of change on the measure that they believe represents a true improvement, or a true lack of improvement, in the patient's status. Frequently, the MCID for the outcome measure is used to distinguish between groups.[15] An example of this would be the CPR to identify patients with acute LBP who respond favorably to manipulation. The investigators chose a 50% improvement on the modified Oswestry Disability Index to indicate a significant change in the patient's disability after manipulation.[11] This represents a fourfold increase over the commonly accepted MCID of 6 points or 12% for this scale.[17]

Once patients have been dichotomized, the categories (e.g., success vs. nonsuccess) are used as the reference standard to compare the individual predictor variables to determine univariate (individual) associations.[5,9] Predictors with statistically significant univariate associations are retained for further analysis. The variables are then entered into a multivariate analysis to determine their contribution to a group of significant predictors. This process is important as occasionally variables with strong individual significance do not contribute to the greater accuracy of a group of predictors. An example of this can be found in the CPR by Flynn et al.[11] In this study, 11 individual variables met the proposed threshold for significance of $p <$ 0.15. Of the 11 variables only five were retained in the final model after multivariate analysis. The final five variables were not necessarily the most significant predictors as indicated by the initial univariate analysis; however, as a group of variables they produced the most significant level of prediction. Thus, the final output of the multivariate analysis is a minimal set of predictor variables that contribute maximal predictive value for the outcome of interest. It is this final set of select predictor variables that comprise the derivation-level CPR.

Although the majority of PT CPRs are derived through prospective cohort studies, there are inherent limitations to this approach with the most important one being the lack of a control group. Without a control group the true treatment effect cannot be established; therefore, although responders are identified, the clinician still does not know if the intervention(s) applied is (are) the most effective for that subgroup. For this reason researchers have recommended the randomized clinical trial (RCT) as the approach of choice due to its controlled manner, ability to reduce bias, and ability to identify treatment effect modifying variables.[18] Regardless of the study design, all agree that the derived CPR should undergo a validation process to confirm the predictive ability of the final variable set.[3–10]

## Validation

As indicated by McGinn et al,[8] the next step in the development of a CPR involves validation of the predictor variables in a narrow and/or broad patient sample. The primary purpose of this step is to confirm that the original predictor variables are neither due to chance or study design, nor are they specific to the patients or setting utilized in the derivation study.[3–9] To accomplish these goals, the validation studies use a new cohort of therapists; a new patient sample derived using the original inclusion/exclusion criteria; and a different treatment setting. Although validation studies utilize various designs, they are most commonly prospective cohort studies or randomized clinical trials. Medical prediction rules such as those that produce risk scores (e.g., deep vein thrombosis, pulmonary embolism) frequently validate the original variables through prospective cohort designs with a different patient population or various combinations of additional diagnostic tests in an attempt to further increase the diagnostic accuracy.[7,8] Validation using a randomized clinical trial is common in the PT literature where interventions are tested and compared either to no intervention or other competing interventions.[9] In this scenario the patient's status on the CPR (i.e., met or not met) is determined prior to randomization. Patients are then randomized using a block design to receive treatment that either matches or does not match the treatment that would be recommended by the results of the CPR. A block design is used to ensure that equal amounts of patients who are positive and negative on the CPR are in both groups to allow for a valid comparison. The subjects then undergo the treatment they were assigned to and their outcome is collected. Once the outcome has been determined, the results are analyzed to determine whether individuals who received a treatment that matched their status on the CPR had superior results compared to those who received unmatched treatment.[9] Randomization also allows for implementation of a competing intervention and in so doing allows the researchers to assess the interaction of the CPR with patients receiving an alternative treatment. Regardless of the approach to validation, this is an extremely important step in the evolutionary process as it helps to improve the clinician's confidence that the results are reproducible and applicable to a larger more diverse patient population.

## Impact Analysis

The third and final step in the CPR development process is the determination of the impact the rule has on clinical practice.[3–9] Reilly and colleagues have suggested the ideal study design for such an analysis would be a randomized clinical trial where the randomization occurs between study sites rather than between treating clinicians.[3] Site randomization enhances the prospects of the rule becoming part of the site's standard operating procedure thus increasing the likelihood of implementation. Upon analysis the researchers should consider the impact of the rule on patient care, its accuracy with or without real-life modifications, and the safety and efficiency of its use. By assessing the multifaceted impact of the rule, the researchers will then be able to determine whether the CPR will truly affect clinical decision making. If the rule is found to affect decision making, it is considered a Level I CPR and may then be referred to as a "clinical decision rule." Practice change is a multifaceted process and can occur for varied reasons thus making the identification of the rule's true impact difficult. Implementation can have many barriers including economic, a lack of resources, rule complexity and its associated cognitive burden, medicolegal fear, and clinician preferences. For this reason, very few prediction rules achieve a Level I status.[3,7,9]

## Summary

Ideally, clinical prediction rules that are routinely used in practice will have undergone full development from derivation to broad validation with a subsequent impact analysis. Some have suggested that rules that have been derived but lack validation (Level IV) are not appropriate for clinical use due to the potential for chance variables and inaccurate findings.[8] In the case of medical prediction rules, the importance of diagnostic accuracy is vital, as the risk of missing a condition may have dire consequences. For this reason, this textbook only includes medical screening CPRs that have undergone broad-based validation (Levels I and II). With regard to PT rules, the risk–benefit ratio is such that if the CPR is followed properly and inclusion/exclusion criteria are applied, the physical therapist is typically dealing with a low-risk intervention and high levels of potential benefit.[9] For this reason, Level IV PT CPRs are included within this text. Although these CPRs may have limited generalizability, sound methodology can allow for the judicious use of their findings as a component of best evidence to guide decision making, particularly in areas where little research exists. It is therefore recommended that clinicians critically analyze derivation-level CPRs to confirm quality and individual patient applicability before implementing them into clinical care.

## Common Methodological Shortcomings of CPR Derivation Studies

### Study Design

The ideal study design to derive DCPRs is the cross-sectional design as it analyzes the effect of variables at one point in time. Longitudinal cohort studies have been proposed as the optimal means to determine factors that may influence the prognosis of an individual with a particular condition over a period of time (PCPR). The goal of an interventional CPR is to identify factors that may influence the treatment effect of an intervention on a subgroup of patients. For this reason, an experimental design such as an RCT has been suggested as the ideal approach to derive these rules. Researchers have indicated that the proper identification of predictor variables for a subgroup of patients can only be achieved through the simultaneous investigation in both an experimental group and a control group.[18] Due to the high cost of RCTs and the large number of subjects required to achieve statistically meaningful results when examining several potential predictor variables, researchers frequently employ cohort-based designs to derive ICPRs. Although this study design does not possess the methodological rigor of the RCT, it begins to identify potential predictor variables and assists in hypothesis generation, making future RCT validation studies more manageable.[18]

## Sample

The astute clinician should begin by analyzing the patient sample to determine whether it is representative of the typical population that would receive the diagnostic test or therapeutic intervention.[8,10] The size of the sample should be adequate to consistently identify predictor variables while also considering the risk of missing an outcome.[9] For this reason researchers have suggested that at least 10–15 patients per potential predictor variable be included in the study.[19] In practice, the determination of the sample size frequently depends on the potential for harm should the patient be misclassified. In situations where the consequences of a missed outcome may be detrimental, the sample size should be large. This is well demonstrated in the medical literature as many CPRs have sample sizes in the thousands.[9,20–25]

Unlike medical diagnostic studies, PT studies generally involve very low risk, thus a lesser degree of precision is acceptable and fewer subjects need to be recruited. Commonly 10–15 subjects per predictor variable in the final CPR model is followed as a recruitment standard.[9,19] Using this suggestion, the recommended recruitment for the Flynn et al.[5] CPR would be 50 subjects as the final CPR contained five variables. Recently a systematic review of PT CPRs has recommended increasing the number of subjects recruited from 10 to 15 per predictor variable in the final model to 10 to 15 subjects per variable entered into multivariate analysis.[26] In this instance Flynn et al.[5] would have a recommended recruitment of 110 subjects as 11 variables were entered into the multivariate analysis. Given that CPRs derived by physical therapists are commonly underpowered, we believe that this recommendation could strengthen the methodological quality of future derivation studies while still maintaining a manageable level of subject recruitment.

## Variable Selection

Beyond sampling, another methodological shortcoming that should be considered includes deriving a prediction rule from a small number of potential predictor variables. It is important to include all the potential predictor variables that may influence the derived rule.[5,9] Variables should be included from the history and physical examination, as well as self-report measures and diagnostic tests. With this being said, it is not always realistic to include a large number of potential predictors as the time required for clinical examination may limit subject participation. For this reason, many initial predictor sets are derived from prior studies, which have identified a prognostic, interventional, or diagnostic link between the variable and the condition or intervention of interest. It is therefore recommended that CPR derivation studies use available evidence to guide and justify the size of the initial set of potential predictor variables.

## Blinding

The importance of blinding is well recognized in other forms of research and the same is true for CPRs. Ideally, the examination will be performed prior to testing on the reference criterion or outcome measures.[3–6,8,10] If the outcome results are not yet known, the examining clinician is inherently blinded; however, if the outcome is known before the exam, it is necessary for the researchers to blind the clinicians from the results to ensure they are not biased. In cases where the outcome is collected after the examination, it is also important to blind the clinician who collects the outcome from the results of the examination to eliminate bias. For this reason, separate clinicians should perform the examination and the intervention. Often in PT research it is very difficult to conceal the intervention from the patient; thus patients are generally aware of the intervention they are receiving, making a double-blinded design rare.

## Outcome Measurement

As mentioned earlier, the outcome measures used to identify predictor variables must possess sufficient validity, reliability, and responsiveness.[3–10] Since the results of the outcome measure are used to determine the "true" outcome for the patient, the validity of the measure is especially important. One concern along these lines is that the determination of change in many of the interventional CPRs is based upon retrospective self-report measures such as Global Rating of Change (GROC) scales. The most commonly utilized GROC scale in the PT literature has been described by Jaeschke et al.[16] It is comprised of a 15-point rating scale ranging from 0 ("about the same") to +7 ("a very great deal better") or −7 ("a very great deal worse"). Other scales do exist, but they have not been frequently utilized in the derivation of PT CPRs.[27,28] Regardless of which global rating scale is used, it should be recognized that they all rely on the patient to determine his or her level of change over a set period of time. Schmitt et al.[29] have demonstrated the potential for recall bias with these measures, as patients may have difficulty recalling their initial status over greater lengths of time. The results, in turn, become a representation of the patient's current status rather than his or her change status. Schmitt et al. therefore suggest caution in utilizing the results of GROC scales as long-term (≥ 4 weeks) outcome measures.[29] They also recommend utilizing multi-item questionnaires to assess functioning across multiple tasks and constructs thus avoiding the potential influence of one difficult task on the patient's perceived level of improvement. Examples of such questionnaires in the PT literature include but are not limited to the Neck Disability Index (NDI),[30] modified Oswestry Disability Index (ODI),[17] Disabilities of the Arm, Shoulder, and Hand (DASH),[31] Lower Extremity Functional Scale (LEFS),[32] and the Patient Specific Functional Status (PSFS).[33]

## Statistical Reporting

Insufficient statistical reporting is another potential flaw found in many CPRs. The most commonly used statistical analysis to derive CPRs is logistic regression. Logistic regressions compare many tests and measures to a dichotomous outcome and determine a parsimonious group of variables that best predict the outcome.[6–9] However, regression analyses can provide other information that is frequently not reported in CPR studies. The statistical significance (expressed as the p-value) of the model derived from the regression analysis can provide readers with the probability that the selected group of variables came about by chance alone. The omission of this statistic precludes the reader from making an accurate judgment on how much he or she should trust the results. Another statistic generated is the $R^2$, or how much variance in the outcome measure the predictor variables account for. This is important as a small $R^2$ value (i.e., they predict a small portion of the variance in the outcome measure) suggests that there may be other variables that could also contribute to prediction of the outcome. Both of these statistics, probability (p) and $R^2$, should be included to allow the physical therapist to more fully and accurately assess the strength of the CPR being considered.[10]

## Reliability of Predictor Tests and Measures

Lastly, accurate determination of change requires not only a blinded evaluator and a valid and responsive outcome measure/reference criterion but also an acceptable level of inter-rater reliability among the tests and measures.[10] Similar to the determination of sample size, the level of acceptable reliability may vary depending upon the CPR and the condition being studied. For example, the reliability of the tests and measures required to diagnose a potentially fatal pulmonary embolism must be very high. On the contrary, the reliability of a measure to determine who will benefit from lumbar stabilization can be lower as the potential for harmful consequences is much less. Reliability therefore lies on a continuum; however, it has been suggested that an acceptable kappa value is $\geq 0.60$, and $\geq 0.70$ is considered an acceptable intra-class correlation coefficient.[10] Reliability statistics should be reported within the body of the CPR. If prior reliability studies do not exist, researchers should perform an internal reliability study to confirm adequate levels among the clinicians involved. A review of the reliability statistics is available in Chapter 3.

# CPR Quality Assessment

The aforementioned list of common methodological shortcomings comprises the overall quality of the CPR study. In determining whether a specific CPR is appropriate and relevant to a particular patient, the clinician must consider the quality of the study's methodology. One might expect an increased level of clinical confidence in the findings of studies that demonstrate high methodological quality and thus consider such CPRs appropriate for implementation into clinical practice. For this reason, the authors have chosen to analyze the quality of derivation-level CPRs to assist the readers in their decision as to whether the rule is appropriate for practice prior to validation. A flow diagram outlining the overall decision process has also been provided in Appendix E.

The first assessment measure that may be used to retrospectively analyze the quality of derivation-level *prognostic* studies was developed by Kuijpers et al.[34] It consists of 18 criteria assessing quality in seven categories: study population, response information, follow-up, treatment, outcome, prognostic factors, and data presentation. Each item is scored as positive, negative, or unclear, with positive scores receiving 1 point, and negative or unclear scores receiving 0 points. The positive scores are added, divided by the total possible points (18), and multiplied by 100 to yield a percentage. Kuijpers et al. recommend an arbitrary cut-off score of at least 60% to indicate a "high-quality" study, and a score of less than 60% to represent a "low-quality" study[34] (**Figure 1.1**).

Recently the tool utilized by Kuijpers et al.[34] has been modified to accommodate analysis of derivation-level *interventional* CPRs. Beneciuk et al.[26] have removed the question regarding response rate and have added an eighth category concerning masking of the outcome assessors and the treating clinicians. The authors noted an intraclass correlation coefficient (ICC) of .73 (95% CI .27–.91), indicating moderate to good inter-rater reliability with this tool.[26] The authors again recommend an arbitrary cut-off score of 60% to indicate a "high-" vs. "low-" quality study (**Figure 1.2**).

Currently, a quality assessment tool for derivation-level *diagnostic* CPRs does not exist, and therefore we have not assigned a quality score to these rules. To help the reader assess the quality of Level IV DCPRs, we have formulated a list of items adapted from prior quality assessment tools, which we believe address many of the elements necessary for a well-designed diagnostic derivation study. The list is intended merely as an assessment guide as it has not undergone the rigors of peer review or a Delphi process for its construction. It is recommended that the clinician critically analyze these CPRs using his or her knowledge of evidence-based practice as well as our table as a guide to determine whether the application of the DCPR is appropriate to his or her specific patient (**Table 1.1**).

**Figure 1.1**
Criteria for assessing
the methodological
quality of prognostic
studies.

A.  Positive if patients were identified at a uniform point (inception cohort) in the course of their disease (first episode, with restriction to duration of symptoms, of shoulder pain in lifetime, or first treated episode of shoulder plain).

B.  Positive if criteria were formulated for at least: age, duration of symptoms, relevant comorbity (i.e., cervical radiculopathy, luxation)/systemic diseases.

C.  Positive if it was described in what setting the patients were recruited (i.e., general practice, hospital, occupational setting).

D.  Positive if the response rate was ≥ 75%.

E.  Positive if information was presented about patient/disease characteristics of responders and non-responders or if there was no selective response.

F.  Positive if a prospective design was used, also positive in case of an historical cohort in which the determinants had been measured before outcome was determined.

G.  Positive if the follow-up period was at least 6 months.

H.  Positive if the total number of participants was ≥ 80% on the last moment of follow-up compared to the number of participants at baseline.

I.  Positive if demographic/clinical information (patient/disease characteristics such as age, sex, and other potential prognostic predictors) was presented for completers and those lost to follow-up/dropouts at the main moment of outcome measurement, or no selective dropouts/lost to follow-up, or no dropouts/lost to follow-up.

J.  Positive if treatment subsequent to inclusion in cohort is fully described or standardized. Also positive in case of no treatment given.

K.  Positive if standardized questionnaires of objective measurements of at least 1 of the following 5 outcome measures were used for each follow-up measurement: pain, general improvement, functional status, general health status, or lost days of work.

L.  Positive if standardized questionnaires or objective measurements were used at baseline for at least 4 of the following 8 potential prognostic factors: age, sex, pain, functional status, duration of complaints, neck complaints, physical workload, or dominant shoulder affected.

M.  Positive if standardized questionnaires or objective measurements were used at baseline of at least 1 of the following 6 potential prognostic factors: depression, somatisation, distress, fear and avoidance, coping strategies, or psychosocial work-related factors (i.e., social support, psychological demands, job decision latitude).

N.  Positive if frequency, percentage or mean, median (Inter Quartile Range), and standard deviation/CI were reported for the most important outcome measures.

O.  Positive if frequency, percentage or mean, median (Inter Quartile Range), and standard deviation/CI were reported for the most important prognostic factors.

P.  Positive if univariate crude estimates were provided for the association of a prognostic factor with outcome.

Q.  Attempt is made to determine a set of prognostic factors with the highest prognostic value.

R.  Positive if the number of cases in the multivariate analysis was at least 10 times the number of independent variables in the analysis (Altman, 1991).

*Source:* Reprinted from
Kuijpers T, van der Windt
D, van der Heijden G,
Bouter LM. Systematic
review of prognostic
cohort studies on
shoulder disorders.
*Pain.* 2005;109:429–
430. Reprinted with
permission from the
International Association
for the Study of Pain.

A. Positive if subjects were identified at an early uniform point (inception cohort) in the course of the condition (first episode, with restriction to duration of symptoms mentioned, of their respective complaint or first physical therapy-related intervention episode for their respective complaint).

B. Positive if criteria were formulated for at least age, duration of symptoms, and relevant comorbidities.

C. Positive if setting in which subjects were treated was described.

D. Positive if information was presented about subject or condition characteristics of responders or nonresponders or if there was no selective process.

E. Positive if a prospective design was used (immediate or same-day follow-up was not considered prospective).

F. Positive if the follow-up period was ≥ 6 months.

G. Positive if the total number of subjects was ≥ 80% at the last moment of the final follow-up compared with the number of subjects at baseline.

H. Positive if demographic or clinical information (subject or condition characteristics, such as age, sex, and other potential prognostic predictors) was presented for subjects completing the study and those lost to follow-up/dropouts at the main moment of baseline outcome measurement, or no selective dropouts/lost to follow-up, or no dropouts/lost to follow-up.

I. Positive if the intervention subsequent to inclusion in a cohort was fully described or standardized (treating clinicians had to adhere to a strict protocol and were not permitted to adjust the intervention on the basis of their independent decision-making processes).

J. Positive if standardized questionnaires or quantitative measurements of at least 1 of the following 5 outcome measures were used for each follow-up measurement: pain, general improvement, functional status, general health status, or lost days of work.

K. Positive if masking of the outcome assessor and treating clinician was achieved. In studies in which self-administered questionnaires were used, masking of the outcome assessor portion of this criterion would be considered acceptable but would have no bearing on the treating clinician status.

L. Positive if standardized questionnaires or objective measurements were used at baseline for at least 4 of the following 6 potential prognostic factors: age, sex, pain, functional status, duration of complaints, or physical work load.

M. Positive if standardized questionnaires or objective measurements were used at baseline for at least 1 of the following 7 potential prognostic factors: depression, somatization, distress, fear-avoidance, coping strategies, anxiety, or psychosocial work-related factors (social support, psychological demands, and job decision latitude).

N. Positive if frequency, percentage, or mean, media, and standard deviation or confidence interval were reported for the most important outcome factors.

O. Positive if frequency, percentage, or mean, media, and standard deviation or confidence interval were reported for the most important prognostic factors.

P. Positive if univariate crude estimates were provided for the association of a prognostic factor with outcome.

Q. Positive if an attempt was made to determine a set of prognostic factors with the highest prognostic value.

R. Positive if the number of cases in the multivariate analysis was at least 10 times the number of independent variables in the multivariate analysis (on the basis of the final clinical prediction rule model, not the initial prospective variables).

**Figure 1.2**
Criteria for assessing the methodological quality of interventional studies.

*Source:* Reprinted from Beneciuk JM, Bishop MD, George SZ. Clinical prediction rules for physical therapy interventions: a systematic review. *Phys Ther*. 2009:89:10–11. Reprinted with permission of the American Physical Therapy Association. This material is copyrighted, and any further reproduction or distribution is prohibited.

**Table 1.1** CPR Quality Assessment of Diagnostic Studies

| Item | Description | Yes | No |
|:---:|:---|:---:|:---:|
| 1 | Inception cohort | | |
| 2 | Prospective and consecutive subjective enrollment | | |
| 3 | Description of setting | | |
| 4 | Description of subject's baseline demographics | | |
| 5 | Clear inclusion/exclusion criteria | | |
| 6 | Recognized valid/reliable reference standard | | |
| 7 | Explanation for predictor variable selection | | |
| 8 | Reliable predictor variables (ICC $\geq$ 0.70; Kappa $\geq$ 0.60) | | |
| 9 | Prospective application of reference standard within a reasonable time frame after the examination | | |
| 10 | Detailed description of positive/negative on reference standard | | |
| 11 | Blinded examiner | | |
| 12 | Blinded interpretation of reference standard | | |
| 13 | Diagnostic accuracy of significant individual predictor variables reported | | |
| 14 | Variables exceeding set cut score for univariate significance entered into regression model | | |
| 15 | Results of regression analysis reported with 95% CIs | | |
| 16 | Statistical significance of the model reported | | |
| 17 | Full description of retained predictor variables presented | | |
| 18 | 10–15 subjects per variable presented in the final clinical prediction rule | | |
| 19 | Were study withdrawals/dropouts < 10% | | |
| | **Total** | | |

Validation of a CPR indicates a higher level of development, and this step is recommended prior to routine implementation of the rule into clinical care. Despite this step the clinician must apply the same critical analysis to these studies as one would to others under consideration for incorporation into patient care, as the mere presence of a validation study does not automatically make the CPR appropriate for use. May and Rosedale[14] have recently adapted a set of proposed quality criteria to retrospectively evaluate *validation* studies of interventional CPRs. The quality measure consists of 10 criteria analyzing the methodological standards of the study. Each item is scored as met (1 point) or not met (0 points). The positive scores are added, divided by the total possible points (10), and multiplied by 100 to yield a percentage. The authors once again recommend an arbitrary cut-off score of 60% or greater to indicate a "high-quality" study, and a score of less than 60% to represent a "low-quality" study. This tool has not currently been validated, and, in our opinion, it requires further expansion to encompass the full quality of a PT-based validation study. However, we have chosen to utilize it as a component of this text in an effort to provide the reader with a means of analyzing the existing PT literature on this topic (**Figure 1.3**).

B. Methodological Standards for Validation of Clinical Prediction Rules
  10. Prospective validation of CPR in a different patient population with different clinicians and in a different setting
  11. Unbiased selection of patients representing a wide spectrum of clinical conditions
  12. Application of rule is adequately taught
  13. Criterion standard applied to all patients to determine true outcome
  14. Accuracy of rule reported—sensitivity, specificity, negative predictive value, positive predictive value, likelihood ratios, with respective 95% confidence intervals
  15. Sample size—at least 10 outcome events per predictor variable in the CPR
  16. Reliability of interpretation of CPR kappa ≥ 0.6
  17. Accuracy of interpretation of CPR
  18. Refinement of CPR, which is then re-validated in a new patient set
  19. Calculation of potential effect if CPR implemented into practice

**Figure 1.3**
Criteria for assessing the methodological quality of interventional validation studies.

*Source:* Adapted from May S, Rosedale R. Prescriptive clinical prediction rules in back pain research: a systematic review. *JMMT.* 2009;17:38. Courtesy of the Journal of Manual and Manipulative Therapy.

## References

1. Sackett DL, Rosenberg WM, Gray JA, Haynes RB, Richardson WS. Evidence based medicine: what it is and what it isn't. *BMJ.* 1996;312:71–72.
2. Brehaut JC, Stiell IG, Visentin L, Graham ID. Clinical decision rules "in the real world": how a widely disseminated rule is used in everyday practice. *Acad Emer Med.* 2005;10:948–956.
3. Reilly BM, Evans AT. Translating clinical research into clinical practice: impact of using prediction rules to make decisions. *Ann Int Med.* 2006;144:201–210.
4. Beattie P, Nelson R. Clinical prediction rules: what are they and what do they tell us? *Aust J Physiother.* 2006;52:157–173.
5. Randolph AG, Guyatt GH, Calvin JE, Doig G, Richardson WS. Understanding articles describing clinical prediction rules. Evidence based medicine in critical care group. *Crit Care Med.* 1998;26:1603–1612.
6. Wasson JH, Sox HC, Neff RK, Goldman L. Clinical prediction rules: application and methodological standards. *NEJM.* 1985;313:793–799.
7. McGinn TG, Guyatt GH, Wyer PC, Naylor C, Stiell IG, Richardson W. Users guide to medical literature: XXII. How to use articles about clinical decision rules. *JAMA.* 2000;284:79–84.
8. Laupacis A, Sekar N, Stiell IG. Clinical prediction rules and suggested modifications of methodological standards. *JAMA.* 1997:277;488–494.
9. Childs JD, Cleland JA. Development and application of clinical prediction rules to improve decision making in physical therapy practice. *Phys Ther.* 2006;86:122–131.
10. Cook CE. Potential pitfall of clinical prediction rules. *JMMT.* 2008:16;69–71.

11.  Flynn T, Fritz J, Whitman J, et al. A clinical prediction rule for classifying patients with low back pain who demonstrate short-term improvement with spinal manipulation. *Spine*. 2002;27:2835–2843.

12.  Fritz JM. Clinical prediction rules in physical therapy: coming of age? *J Orthop Sports Phys Ther*. 2009;39:159–161.

13.  Stiell IG, Wells GA. Methodological standards for the development of clinical decision rules in emergency medicine. *Ann Emerg Med*. 1999;33:437–447.

14.  May S, Rosedale R. Prescriptive clinical prediction rules in back pain research: a systematic review. *JMMT*. 2009;17:36–45.

15.  Resnik L, Dobrzykowski E. Guide to outcome measurement for patients with low back syndrome. *J Orthop Sports Phys Ther*. 2003;33:307–318.

16.  Jaeschke R, Singer J, Guyatt GH. Measurement of health status. Ascertaining the minimal clinically important difference. *Control Clin Trials*. 1989;10:407–415.

17.  Fritz JM, Irrgang JJ. A comparison of a modified Oswestry low back pain disability pain questionnaire and the Quebec back pain disability scale. *Phys Ther*. 2001;81:776–788.

18.  Hancock M, Herbert RD, Maher CG. A guide to interpretation of studies investigating subgroups of responders to physical therapy interventions. *Phys Ther*. 2009;89:698–704.

19.  Concato J, Feinstein AR, Holford TR. The risk of determining risk with multivariate methods. *Ann Int Med*. 1993;118:201–210.

20.  Stiell IG, Greenberg GH, McKnight RD, Nair RC, McDowell I, Worthington JR. A study to develop clinical decision rules for the use of radiography in acute ankle injuries. *Ann Emerg Med*. 1992;21:384–390.

21.  Stiell IG, Greenberg GH, Wells GA, et al. Derivation of a decision rule for the use of radiography in acute knee injuries. *Ann Emerg Med*. 1995;26:405–413.

22.  Stiell IG, Wells GA, Vandemheen KL, et al. The Canadian C-spine rule for radiography in alert and stable trauma patients. *JAMA*. 2001;286:1841–1848.

23.  Stiell IG, Wells GA, Vandemheen KL, et al. The Canadian CT head rule for patients with minor head injury. *Lancet*. 2001;357:1391–1396.

24.  Wells PS, Anderson DR, Rodger M, et al. Derivation of a simple clinical model to categorize patient's probability of pulmonary embolism: increasing the models utility with the SimpliRed D-dimer. *Thromb Haemost*. 2000;83:416–420.

25.  Mower WR, Hoffman JR, Herbert M, Wolfson AB, Pollack CV, Zucker MI. Developing a decision instrument to guide computed tomographic imaging of blunt head injury patients. *J Trauma*. 2005;59:954–959.

26.  Beneciuk JM, Bishop MD, George SZ. Clinical prediction rules for physical therapy interventions: a systematic review. *Phys Ther*. 2009:89:114–124.

27.  Dworkin RH, Turk DC, Farrar JT, et al. Core outcome measures for chronic pain clinical trials. IMMPACT recommendations. *Pain*. 2005;113:9–19.

28.  Stewart M, Maher CG, Refshauge KM, Bogduk N, Nicholas M. Responsiveness of pain and disability measures for chronic whiplash. *Spine*. 2007;32:580–585.

29.  Schmitt J, Di Fabio RP. The validity of prospective and retrospective global change criterion measures. *Arch Phys Med Rehabil*. 2005;86:2270–2276.

30.  Vernon H, Mior S. The neck disability index: a study of reliability and validity. *J Manipulative Physiol Ther*. 1991;14:409–415.

31. Hudak PL, Amadio PC, Bombardier C. The Upper Extremity Collaborative Group (UECG). Development of an upper extremity outcome measure: the DASH (disabilities of the arm, shoulder and hand). *Am J Ind Med*. 1996;29:602–608.

32. Binkley JM, Stratford PW, Lott SA, Riddle DL. The Lower Extremity Functional Scale (LEFS): scale development, measurement properties, and clinical application. North American Orthopaedic Rehabilitation Research Network. *Phys Ther*. 1999;79:371–383.

33. Stratford P, Gill C, Westaway M, Binkley J. Assessing disability and change on individual patients: a report of a patient specific measure. *Physiotherapy Canada*. 1995;47:258–263.

34. Kuijpers T, van der Windt D, van der Heijden G, Bouter LM. Systematic review of prognostic cohort studies on shoulder disorders. *Pain*. 2004;109:420–431.

# CHAPTER 2

# HOW TO USE THIS BOOK

The purpose of this book is to serve as a clinical resource and reference manual for a collection of clinical prediction rules pertinent to the outpatient, orthopedic physical therapist. This book is intended to augment clinical decision making in areas where further research is required. CPRs should not be used in isolation while making decisions, but rather as one component of the larger clinical decision-making process. We believe that when considered within the larger context of evidence-based practice, prediction rules can be very helpful in uncovering associations that unstructured clinical observation might otherwise miss. We therefore recommend that one considers these CPRs along with the current existing evidence, patient preferences, and clinical experience when reaching clinical decisions. When used in this manner, CPRs strengthen clinical decision making.

As autonomous practitioners with the potential to be frontline health care providers, it is the physical therapist's responsibility to recognize conditions that may require a medical examination. For this reason, we provide a large section on diagnostic imaging prediction rules as well as others to help screen for conditions beyond the scope of physical therapy treatment. The rules that we provide include those that contain subjective and/or objective variables that can be obtained within a physical therapy examination or treatment session. Rules that contain variables that cannot currently be obtained by physical therapists have not been included in this book. We therefore do not claim to provide an exhaustive list of CPRs, but rather those that we feel are the most pertinent to the practicing orthopedic physical therapist.

The book has been divided into two primary sections. The first section includes prediction rules to assist physical therapists with screening for conditions that will require referral to another medical practitioner. The rules have been separated based upon imaging type and body systems. They have also been further subdivided into diagnostic or prognostic categories. Section two includes the musculoskeletal prediction rules that are most pertinent to physical therapists. They are divided into body regions and then subdivided into the individual joints. Lastly, to help improve

Health Sciences Library
University of Saskatchewan Libraries
Room B205 Health Sciences Building
107 WIGGINS ROAD
SASKATOON, SK S7N 5E5 CANADA

the utility of the reference manual we have listed the rules as diagnostic, prognostic, or interventional.

Each individual prediction rule has been organized to provide clinicians with readily available information to help determine whether it applies to the patient sitting before them. Immediately after the title, information regarding the primary category of the rule (diagnostic, prognostic, or interventional) as well as the level of development (IV–I) is listed. For Level IV prognostic or interventional CPRs, a score is provided to indicate the methodological quality of the rule. Prognostic CPRs contain a quality assessment score reflective of the tool utilized by Kuijpers et al.,[1] and interventional CPRs contain a quality assessment score indicative of the tool adapted by Beneciuk et al.[2] Individual item scoring for each CPR can be found in Appendices A, B, and D. Level IV diagnostic-level CPRs do not contain a quality score because an analytical tool currently does not exist; however, we propose a tool to help guide the quality analysis of these rules that can be found in Appendix C. The header section of each rule is followed by a "blink" box that provides a definition of "positive" for that particular CPR as well as the defining statistics. Next, the reader is introduced to the parsimonious set of predictor variables. Finally, a summative "clinical bottom line" providing an explanation of the findings and their potential clinical impact completes the first page. The next page(s) contain(s) the specifics of the clinical tests, measures, and interventions, with descriptions and pictures as well as a brief summary of the study's background information. This information includes the inclusion/exclusion criteria, patient demographic information, a definition of positive or "success," as well as the validation and impact studies that have been published. The summary of background information is not meant to replace the original works, and readers are strongly encouraged to obtain and read the studies to have a more complete understanding of the CPR, which will further strengthen clinical decision making. A summary of the validation studies has been included to provide a more informed decision regarding the similarity of a particular patient to the population from which the CPR was tested. PT intervention validation studies also contain a quality score reflective of the tool utilized by May and Rosedale as a component of the validation synopsis to provide the reader with further information upon which to base clinical decisions.[3] Lastly, a full list of available references applicable to each rule is provided. Although the above information will provide readers with the means to determine whether the CPR is appropriate for the patient sitting before them, it is recommended that they refer to the original study for the full details before implementing the findings.

The primary aim of this reference manual is to provide a readily available list of clinical prediction rules. We have arranged the data to maximize clinical utility as well as provide pertinent information so that clinicians can determine whether the rule and its outcomes are appropriate for their patient scenario. It is important to remember that CPRs are not a substitute for decision making; rather they are tools to help guide the decision-making process, whether diagnostic, prognostic, or interventional. By combining experience, patient's values, and the best current evidence, which includes prediction rules, clinicians can make informed decisions as to the most effective and efficient way to care for their patients.

## References

1. Kuijpers T, van der Windt D, van der Heijden G, Bouter LM. Systematic review of prognostic cohort studies on shoulder disorders. *Pain*. 2004;109:420–431.
2. Beneciuk JM, Bishop MD, George SZ. Clinical prediction rules for physical therapy interventions: a systematic review. *Phys Ther*. 2009:89:114–124.
3. May S, Rosedale R. Prescriptive clinical prediction rules in back pain research: a systematic review. *JMMT*. 2009;17:36–45.

# STATISTICS

One of the advantages of using CPRs is that the statistical investigation of the complex interaction of variables in clinical decision making can uncover relationships that may not otherwise have been discovered. To assist the clinician in evaluating and interpreting the growing body of literature related to development, validation, and analysis of CPRs, we include a brief review of the pertinent statistics. We first present statistical parameters commonly used in diagnostic accuracy studies, follow with measures of reliability, and finally provide an introduction to common statistical analyses used in the derivation of a CPR. A complete review of these statistical methods is beyond the scope of this book and is available elsewhere.[1–4]

# Common Statistical Parameters in Diagnostic Accuracy Studies

The results of clinical prediction rules are frequently reported using diagnostic accuracy statistics. This would seem obvious for DCPRs as there is a dichotomous reference standard (disease present, disease absent); however, the use of these statistics in the development of ICPRs and PCPRs may be less apparent. For ICPRs, the predictor variables are compared to the post-intervention outcome of the patient, and, in the case of PCPRs, the predictor variables are compared to the patient's outcome at predetermined post-intervention time intervals. In essence, the diagnosis the therapist is trying to make in these cases is not the presence or absence of pathology; rather the goal is to predict the patient's outcome. For this reason, the statistics most commonly reported in CPRs are *sensitivity*, *specificity*, *likelihood ratios*, and the *associated confidence intervals*.[5]

## Sensitivity and Specificity

Sensitivity (Sn) and specificity (Sp) are statistical parameters that describe the measurement validity of a diagnostic test with regard to the relationship between the findings on the test compared to the findings on the reference standard. In this context, the diagnostic test is usually the clinical test under investigation and the reference standard (sometimes called the gold standard) is what is used to determine the true diagnosis. In the case of prognostic and interventional CPRs, the reference standard includes the patient's outcome either after treatment or after a designated period of time. In a diagnostic accuracy study (or a CPR), there are four possible results from the comparison of the diagnostic test to the reference standard. These are often presented in a 2×2 contingency table, as seen in **Table 3.1**. The four possible results are (1) True Positive (when the diagnostic test is positive and the reference standard is positive); (2) True Negative (when the diagnostic test is negative and the reference standard is negative); (3) False Positive (when the diagnostic test is positive, but the reference standard is actually negative); and (4) False Negative (when the diagnostic test is negative, but the reference standard is actually positive).[6] Sensitivity and specificity are the proportion of correct tests among individuals with and without the condition and are derived from the results of the 2×2 contingency table. Sensitivity is the proportion of patients with the condition (as defined by a positive test on the reference standard) who tested positive on the diagnostic test. Mathematically this can be calculated from the left side of the 2×2 table. As seen in Table 3.1, sensitivity is equal to the number of true positives divided by the sum of true positives and false negatives. Note that sensitivity does not consider the number of false negatives or true positives. Specificity is the

**Table 3.1** 2×2 Contingency Table for Diagnostic Tests with Sensitivity and Specificity Calculations

|  | Reference Standard Positive | Reference Standard Negative |
|---|---|---|
| **Diagnostic Test Positive** | true positive | false positive |
| **Diagnostic Test Negative** | false negative | true negative |
|  | **Sensitivity** | **Specificity** |
|  | $\dfrac{\text{true positives}}{\text{true positives + false negatives}}$ | $\dfrac{\text{true negatives}}{\text{true negatives + false positives}}$ |

proportion of patients without the condition (as defined by a negative test on the reference standard) who tested negative on the diagnostic test. This can be calculated from the left side of the 2×2 table by dividing the number of true negatives by the sum of true negatives and false positives. Specificity does not take into account true positives or false negatives. Sensitivity and specificity are generally reported as a percentage or a decimal.[6] For example, the sensitivity and specificity of the Canadian Cervical Spine Rules are 100% and 43%, respectively (or this can be written 1.0 and 0.43, respectively).[7]

Based on the definitions above, the clinical utility of these tests is counterintuitive. With sensitivity defined as the "proportion of patients with the condition who tested positive on the test," one would think that a test with high sensitivity will identify patients with the condition of interest. However, sensitivity is calculated only from true positives and false negatives. A test with high sensitivity will have many true positives and few false negatives, but the false positive rate is not taken into account for this statistic. Therefore, we cannot be certain that a positive test is a true positive or a false positive; however, the fact that tests with high sensitivity have few false negatives means that if a highly sensitive test is negative, there is a high probability that the patient does not have the condition of interest.[6] For this reason highly sensitive tests are best used to rule out a condition and are ideal for screening patients for pathology that would require medical referral. The Canadian Cervical Spine Rule is a good example of this.[7] It has a sensitivity of virtually 100%, so if a patient is negative on the rule, the probability of a fracture of the cervical spine is effectively zero and radiographic evaluation is not necessary. Conversely, a highly specific test is better used to rule in a condition because it has a low false-positive rate. If it is positive, there is a high probability that the patient does have the condition of interest.[6] In the example above, the specificity of the Canadian Cervical

Spine Rule is 43%, which is low and therefore an unacceptable test to rule in a fracture without radiography. Due to the potential consequences of a missed fracture, in the absence of a negative response, radiography is therefore warranted.[7] A commonly used mnemonic to remember the purpose of each test is SpPIn (**Sp**ecificity, **P**ositive test to rule **In**) and SnNOut (**Sen**sitivity, **N**egative test to rule **Out**).[8]

In the context of interpreting CPRs, one of the more useful statistical measures is sensitivity, particularly in CPRs that physical therapists use in screening patients for medical referral. A negative result on a highly sensitive CPR, such as the Canadian Cervical Spine Rule, suggests that the clinician can be confident that there is a high probability that no cervical spine fractures are present and treatment may be initiated. CPRs used for screening do not require a high level of specificity as their primary purpose is to ensure that a condition is not missed. If a potentially serious condition cannot be ruled out due to a positive result on a sensitive CPR, a referral to the appropriate medical provider would be the prudent course of action.

Despite the ability of sensitivity and specificity values to help guide clinical decision making, it is important to remember that they are point estimates and may involve wide variations in the actual findings (wide confidence intervals).[9] Such variations weaken the clinical utility of these values, and it is therefore recommended that other statistics, which consider both sensitivity and specificity, be considered. One such statistic is the likelihood ratio.

## Likelihood Ratios

Likelihood ratios (LR) are additional measures of the validity of a test (i.e., DCPRs) or cluster of predictor variables (i.e., ICPRs or PCPRs) and are derived from sensitivity and specificity values. However, unlike sensitivity and specificity values, which create a shift in direction only, likelihood ratios quantify both the direction and magnitude of the shift in probability that an individual will be positive or negative on the reference standard.[6] Additionally, Sn and Sp values produce a dichotomous, single-level outcome, where LRs can produce multiple outcome levels. Finally, because LRs are calculated from sensitivity and specificity, which do not fluctuate depending on prevalence, LRs are also not prevalence dependent and thus are not subject to inflation due to the patient sample.[6]

Likelihood ratios are positive or negative in direction. A positive (+)LR indicates the shift in probability that a patient who is positive on the diagnostic test would also be positive on the reference standard. Conversely, a negative (−)LR indicates the shift in probability that a patient who is negative on the diagnostic test would also be negative on the reference standard. LRs are reported as a single number, with a value of 1 indicating the test result does not produce a shift in the posttest probability of the presence or absence of the condition. Positive LRs that are greater than 1 describe an increasing post-test probability that patients who test positive will possess the condition of interest, and negative LRs less than 1 describe an increasing posttest probability that patients who test negative will not possess the condition.[6] Guidelines for interpreting the magnitude of the shift in probability have been suggested and are presented in **Table 3.2**.

Positive LRs of 1–2 are considered small and rarely important shifts in probability for the condition/response. Positive LRs of 2–5 are considered

**Table 3.2** A Guide to Interpretation of Likelihood Ratio (LR) Values

| Positive LR | Negative LR | Interpretation |
|-------------|-------------|----------------|
| > 10 | < 0.1 | Generate large and often conclusive shifts in probability |
| 5–10 | 0.1–0.2 | Generate moderate shifts in probability |
| 2–5 | 0.2–0.5 | Generate small, but sometimes important, shifts in probablity |
| 1–2 | 0.5–1 | Alter probability to a small, and rarely important, degree |

*Source:* Reprinted from Fritz JM, Wainner RS. Examining diagnostic tests: an evidence-based perspective. *Phys Ther.* 2001; 81:1536. Reprinted with permission of the American Physical Therapy Association. This material is copyrighted, and any further reproduction or distribution is prohibited.

small, but sometimes important shifts in probability for the condition/response. Positive LRs of 5–10 indicate moderate and meaningful shifts in probability for the condition/response. Finally, positive LRs greater than 10 are large and often conclusive shifts in probability for having the condition. Conversely, negative LRs of 0.5–1 are considered small and rarely important. Negative LRs of 0.2–0.5 are considered small and sometimes important. Negative LRs of 0.1–0.2 are considered moderate and meaningful shifts in probability. Negative LRs of less than 0.1 indicate large and often conclusive shifts in probability for not having the condition.[6,10]

Ideally all clinical prediction rules would have positive LRs of greater than 10 or negative LRs of less than 0.1 to make clinical decision making clear. However, it is not uncommon for a CPR derivation study to find a small or moderate LR (i.e., +LRs = 2–10 or –LRs = 0.5–0.1), as demonstrated by Sutlive et al.[11] in which +LR of 4 was found for patients with patellofemoral pain who may benefit from orthotics. A +LR of 4 creates a small shift in posttest probability; however, the clinical significance of this shift is uncertain. Therefore, clinicians must combine the probability shift of the LR with an estimate of the pretest probability that the patient has the condition of interest and will respond to the treatment of interest, or will have the outcome of interest. Estimates of the pretest probability can be based on historical and demographic data, prevalence rates, and previous experiences with patients of similar clinical presentation.[6] In the example above, if a clinician is going to treat a patient with patellofemoral pain and his or her past experience treating a similar patient with orthotics produced good results, the pretest probability for a similar response would be relatively high; perhaps a 60% chance of benefiting from orthotics. If the examination findings meet the criteria of the CPR, the physical therapist can use a tool called a Fagan's nomogram (**Figure 3.1**) to combine the

**Figure 3.1**
Fagan's nomogram.

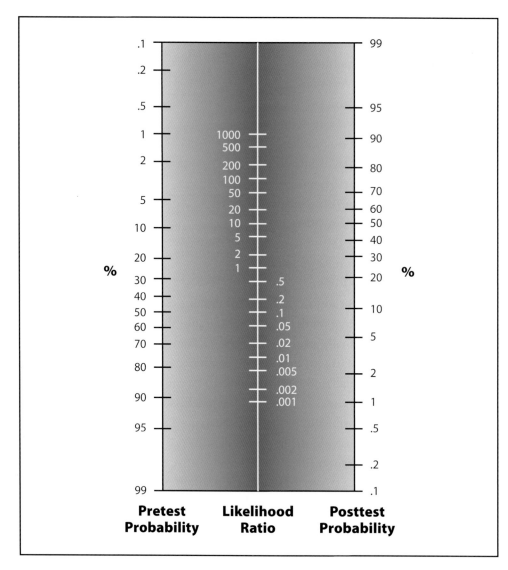

*Source:* Reprinted from Fagan TJ. Nomogram for Baye's theorem. *N Engl J Med.* 1975;293:257. Reprinted with permission from the Massachusetts Medical Society. This material is copyrighted © 1975 Massachusetts Medical Society. All rights reserved.

pretest probability with the positive LR to determine the posttest probability for successful intervention.[12] Electronic versions of Fagan's nomogram are also available for rapid clinical use (http://www.cebm.net/index.aspx?o=1161).[13] In the example above, a pretest probability of 60% combined with a positive LR of 4 yields a post-test probability of ~85%. Therefore, the clinician may go forward with the orthotic intervention despite the small positive LR.

As indicated above, the estimation of pretest probability is subject to the influence of multiple considerations. Despite this, the clinician must consider the full context of the decision making. As many interventions utilized by physical therapists carry low levels of risk, a more general estimate of pretest probability, based upon experience rather than epidemiological data, may be reasonable. If this estimate is combined with a large and conclusive shift in posttest probability (+LR > 10), the therapist should feel comfortable and confident applying the treatment. If the pretest probability is low or the likelihood ratio is small to moderate, the therapist may still choose to implement the treatment if a more evidence-based option does not exist.

## Confidence Intervals

The sensitivity, specificity, and LR values generated from studies are calculated only from the study sample and are therefore only point *estimates* of the true value. Confidence intervals (CIs) describe how precise these estimates are. The most commonly reported CI is the 95% CI, which indicates the range of values that we can be 95% certain that the true value falls within.[14,15] In general, it is favorable to have a 95% CI that encompasses a narrow range of estimates. An example of a CPR with a narrow CI is the sensitivity of the Canadian Cervical Spine Rules, which has a sensitivity of 1.0 and a 95% CI of .98 to 1.0.[7] This means that we can be 95% certain that the true sensitivity of this cluster lies between .98 and 1.0, which is very good due to the narrow width of the interval. Conversely, a wide 95% CI makes us less confident in the reported point estimate.[14,15] An example of a wide 95% CI is the diagnostic CPR for cervical radiculopathy.[16] If a patient meets all four criteria, the positive LR is 30.3 (i.e., the point estimate), which indicates a large shift in probability that the patient has cervical radiculopathy. However, the 95% CI is 1.7 to 538.2, which indicates the potential for a shift in probability ranging from small and rarely important (i.e., 1.7) to large and conclusive (i.e., 538.2).[6,10] The breadth of the CI is dependent upon, among other things, the number of subjects included in the analysis and the amount of variance in the sample with fewer subjects and greater variance contributing to a broader CI.[1,14] The positive LR for patients with cervical radiculopathy who meet all four criteria on the CPR is 30.3. However, of the 73 subjects comprising the sample, only 16 were positive for radiculopathy on the reference criterion.[16] Due to the small number of subjects positive on the rule, the resultant CI was wide (95% CI: 1.7–538.2). When three of the four criteria were met, the 95% CI for the positive LR (6.1) is considerably more narrow (95% CI: 2.0–18.6), indicating greater precision of the estimate. In principle, clinicians judge their degree of confidence in the results based on the 95% CI, but how they apply the results to clinical decision making should be based on the consequences involved with making an incorrect decision. In the case of the Canadian Cervical Spine Rules there could be potentially serious consequences associated with unidentified cervical fracture; therefore, clinicians should use tests or CPRs with narrow confidence intervals indicating precise estimates. An imprecise estimate would be unacceptable given the consequences of missing a cervical spine fracture. On the other hand, given that there are few, and minor, risks associated with initiating conservative management of cervical radiculopathy when it is not present, clinicians can apply the results of a less precise estimate without increasing risk to the patient.[1,6]

## Reliability

### Intraclass Correlation Coefficient

Intraclass correlation coefficient (ICC) is a measure of reliability that can be used for continuous data. The output of ICCs range from 0.00 (indicating no agreement) to 1.00 (indicating perfect agreement). Guidelines for the interpretation of these numbers have suggested that values above 0.75 indicate good reliability and those below 0.75 indicate poor/moderate reliability.[1]

### Kappa

The kappa ($\kappa$) statistic is another measure of reliability, which is primarily used for categorical data (nominal and ordinal). It is similar to percent agreement; however, percent agreement usually leads to inflated reliability numbers because chance agreements are included in the overall calculation. The kappa statistic accounts for chance agreements, thus providing a more accurate estimate of reliability. The $\kappa$ value can range from −1.00 (indicating agreement that is worse than chance) to 1.00 (indicating perfect agreement).[1,17] While many scales exist to interpret the level of agreement proposed by the kappa statistic, these scales are merely guidelines as the amount of reliability necessary for a particular test, intervention, and so on exist along a continuum and may vary depending on the clinical scenario. Despite the inability of the $\kappa$ statistic to stand alone in guiding decision making, a threshold value of $\geq 0.60$ has been suggested as a methodological standard for CPRs in an attempt to eliminate error.[18]

## Statistics Used in CPR Derivation

### T-Test and Chi-Square

The t-test and chi-square are fundamental tests for differences between two groups. The t-test is a parametric statistical test used with normally distributed continuous data, whereas the chi-square is a nonparametric statistical test for use with categorical data. These statistical analyses test for differences between group means (t-test) or frequency of observations (chi-square), and the within-group variation of the scores determine the probability that the observed difference between groups is due to chance.[1] The most useful output of both tests is the "p-value," which describes the likelihood that the difference in the means is due to chance. The p-value can range from 0 to 1.0; the cutoff point for a meaningful p-value is determined after conducting the initial univariate analysis. Generally investigators set a p-value of less than or equal to 0.05 as the threshold (significance level) of chance they are willing to accept. This means that there is less than a 5% chance that the observed differences are due to chance, and a 95% chance that the results are due to a true difference.[1] Although the p-value is typically, and arbitrarily, set at 0.05, different levels can be chosen depending on the purpose of the study. Some investigators set a more conservative significance level of 0.01, meaning that the investigators are willing to accept a 1% chance that the observed differences may be due to chance. On the other hand, other studies such as CPR derivations frequently use a more liberal significance level, as high as 0.15. This liberal significance level is chosen to ensure that potential predictor variables are not excluded from the subsequent logistic regression analysis.[5]

## Receiver Operating Characteristic Curve

A receiver operating characteristic (ROC) curve is a graphical representation used to investigate the relationship between true positives and false positives across the range of scores on the diagnostic test. ROC curves are used to determine the score that maximizes true positives and minimizes false positives, and thus, provide the score at which the test is most diagnostic, predictive, or prognostic.[1] Determination of cutoff scores is the focus of this discussion as it pertains to the development of CPRs. An example of this is in the CPR for benefit from lumbopelvic manipulation for low back pain.[19] One of the predictor variables is duration of symptoms. For this information to be useful for clinicians, we need to know at what point the duration of symptoms is most predictive of benefit from manipulation. To do this the sensitivity and specificity for each possible cutoff value is calculated, then each cutoff point is plotted on a graph with its sensitivity on the *y*-axis and 1-specificity plotted on the *x*-axis. The point at the upper left of the graph represents the point that is the best overall cutoff score and is most frequently used. In the case of the lumbar manipulation CPR, using the ROC curve, it was determined that symptom duration of 16 days or fewer is predictive of success with manipulation.

## Multivariate Analysis

### Logistic Regression in CPR Derivation

A common statistical analysis used in the derivation of a CPR is logistic regression. Logistic regression analysis consists of three basic steps: identification of candidate predictor variables; determination of cutoff scores; and determination of the predictor variable cluster. Initially, each predictor variable is individually compared to the outcome to see whether there is a univariate relationship using t-test and chi square analyses as described previously. Investigators commonly use a liberal significance level (generally $p < 0.1$) to ensure all variables with potential predictive power are not excluded. Variables that meet the $p < 0.1$ significance level are retained for further analysis, and the others are discarded.[5] Next, the ROC curve is analyzed, as described previously, to determine the cutoff score for each continuous variable that is most diagnostic, prognostic, or predictive. The final step is to determine the cluster of variables that best predicts the outcome, which is done using regression analysis. A complete description of regression analysis is beyond the scope of this book; however, it can consider multiple variables and determine the relative contributions of each variable on the outcome, and it can also determine how groups of variables contribute to the outcome, using a regression equation.[2–4] For CPRs, the most frequently used type of regression analysis is logistic regression because CPR studies frequently use a dichotomous outcome and the predictor variables can be continuous or categorical. Furthermore, logistic regression can be run using the full set of independent variables or using a stepwise procedure.[1] The result is a parsimonious group of variables that describes the relationship to the outcome in terms of sensitivity, specificity, likelihood ratios, and probability of success.

### Recursive Partitioning

Recursive partitioning is a nonparametric discriminate analysis technique that repeatedly stratifies subjects in a study into smaller and smaller subgroups based on characteristics that predict the desired outcome.[2] This technique works best when the outcome is dichotomous, as it is in most prediction rules (i.e., the subject responds to treatment or does not for intervention CPRs; the subject has the condition or does not for diagnostic CPRs; the subject has persistent disability or does not for prognostic CPRs). The repeated subgrouping is achieved by taking the initial set of patients and comparing the discriminate ability of each possible predictor variable based on maximizing the change of an "index of diversity." The predictor variable that best discriminates between the two outcomes is selected. Next, the process is repeated for the two groups that were just created, again comparing the group to each of the predictor variables and selecting the one that maximized the "index of diversity." This iterative process continues creating a tree diagram until a predetermined stopping point is reached, which is selected based on the total number of stratifications that will occur (more stratifications may make a more complex CPR) and the cost of misclassification associated with the rule. The "index of diversity" is based on a measure of the amount of endpoint diversity within the group being examined and takes into account prior probabilities for each endpoint category and the relative costs of misclassification to either category.[2] The results of the analysis are the significant predictor variables that make the CPR, and the sensitivity, specificity, and likelihood ratios can then be calculated to describe the rule.

Due to the repeated stratification into smaller subgroups, one disadvantage of this approach is the extremely large sample size necessary to maintain a sufficient number of subjects for analysis. Thus clinicians must confirm adequate power when analyzing studies utilizing this approach.

## References

1. Portney LG, Watkins MP. *Foundations of Clinical Research: Applications to Practice*. Norwalk, CT: Appleton & Lange; 1993.
2. Cook EF, Goldman L. Empiric comparison of multivariate analytic techniques: advantages and disadvantages of recursive partitioning analysis. *J Chron Dis*. 1984;37:721–731.
3. Guyatt G, Walter S, Shannon H, Cook D, Jaeschke R, Heddle N. Basic statistics for clinicians: 4. Correlation and regression. *Can Med Assoc J*. 1995;152:497–504.
4. Rudy TE, Kubinski JA, Boston JR. Multivariate and repeated measurements: a primer. *J Critical Care*. 1992;7:30–41.
5. Childs JD, Cleland JA. Development and application of clinical prediction rules to improve decision making in physical therapy practice. *Phys Ther*. 2006;86:122–131.
6. Fritz JM, Wainner RS. Examining diagnostic tests: an evidence-based perspective. *Phys Ther*. 2001;81:1546–1564.
7. Stiell IG, Wells GA, Vandemheen KL, et al. The Canadian C-spine rule for radiography in alert and stable trauma patients. *JAMA*. 2001;286:1841–1848.
8. Sackett D, Haynes R, Guyatt G, Tugwell P. *Clinical Epidemiology: A Basic Science for Clinical Medicine*. Boston: Little Brown; 1992.
9. Hegedus EJ, Stern B. Beyond SpPIN and SnNOUT: considerations with dichotomous tests during assessment of diagnostic accuracy. *JMMT*. 2009;17:E1–E5.
10. Jaeschke R, Guyatt GH, Sackett DL. Users' guide to the medical literature, III: how to use an article about a diagnostic test, B: what are the results and will they help me in caring for my patients? *JAMA*. 1994;271:703–707.
11. Sutlive TG, Mitchell SD, Maxfield SN, et al. Identification of individuals with patellofemoral pain whose symptoms improved after a combined program of foot orthosis use and modified activity: a preliminary investigation. *Phys Ther*. 2004;84:49–61.
12. Fagan TJ. Nomorgram for Baye's theorem. *N Engl J Med*. 1975;293:257.
13. Centre for Evidence Based Medicine. Interactive nomogram [Web page]. Available at: http://www.cebm.net/index.aspx?o=1161. Accessed May 16, 2009.
14. Noteboom TJ, Allison SC, Cleland JA, Whitman JW. A primer on selected aspects of evidence-based practice relating to questions of treatment, part 2: interpreting results, application to clinical practice, and self-evaluation. *J Orthop Sports Phys Ther*. 2008;38:485–501.
15. Sim J, Reid N. Statistical inference by confidence intervals: issues of interpretation and utilization. *Phys Ther*. 1999;79:186–195.

16. Wainner RS, Fritz JM, Irrgang JJ, Boninger ML, Delitto A, Allison S. Reliability and diagnostic accuracy of the clinical examination and patient self-report measures for cervical radiculopathy. *Spine*. 2003;28:52–62.

17. Sim J, Wright CC. The kappa statistic in reliability studies: use, interpretation and sample size requirement. *Phys Ther*. 2005;85:257–268.

18. Laupacis A, Sekar N, Stiell IG. Clinical prediction rules: a review and suggested modifications of methodological standards. *JAMA*. 1997;277:488–494.

19. Flynn T, Fritz J, Whitman J, et al. A clinical prediction rule for classifying patients with low back pain who demonstrate short-term improvement with spinal manipulation. *Spine*. 2002;27:2835–2843.

*Validation/Impact Analysis*

- Prospective refinement and validation of the rule. Refinement included dropping age as a predictor. Validation found that the refined rule had a Sn of 1.0 (95% CI 0.97–1.0) and a Sp of 0.49 (95% CI 0.44–0.54) for ankle fracture. Additionally, its implementation would have led to a 34% decrease in the use of radiography.[2]
- Prospective impact analysis where one ED implemented the Ottawa Ankle Rules (OAR) and the other did not. In the OAR ED, there was a 28% decrease in ankle radiography, patients spent ~36 minutes less waiting in the ED, medical costs were $111 less, and there was no difference in patient satisfaction. In addition, sensitivity for detecting ankle fracture was maintained at 1.0 (95% CI 0.95–1.0).[3]
- Prospective external validation of the rule as used by physicians and triage nurses. For physicians, Sn was 1.0 and Sp was 0.19. For triage nurses, Sn was 0.9 and Sp was 0.1. Application of the rules would have led to a 19% reduction in use of midfoot and ankle radiographs.[4]
- Prospective multicenter validation. Results found a Sn of 0.93 and a Sp of 0.11. Authors concluded that the rule's false negative rate was too high to recommend implementation in New Zealand EDs.[5]
- Cost-effectiveness analysis of the OAR comparing the decision rule with current practice. Results found that in the United States savings ranged from $614,226 to $3,145,910 per 100,000 patients. In Canada savings were CAN$730,145 per 100,000 patients.[6]
- Prospective validation of the rule with every subject examined receiving a radiograph. Results indicated a Sn of 0.95 and a Sp of 0.16 for ankle fractures and a Sn of 0.93 and a Sp of 0.12 for midfoot fractures.[7]
- Multicenter impact analysis assessing use of radiography, ED wait times, cost of treatment, and missed fractures before and after implementing the OAR in eight hospitals. Results indicated significant decreases in radiography use, ED wait times, and cost of treatment without increase in missed fractures after implementation of the OAR.[8]
- Multicenter impact analysis of implementation of the OAR in France. Results indicated that radiograph use decreased by 22.4% after implementation.[9]
- Prospective evaluation in a sports medicine population. Results indicated that the rule had a Sn of 1.0 and a Sp of 0.4 and would have decreased radiography use by 34%.[10]

- Pooled analysis from seven studies found that the OAR had a Sn of 0.97 and a Sp ranging from 0.3 to 0.6.[11]
- Prospective validation in children 1–15 years old. Results indicate that the OAR had a Sn of 0.98 and a Sp of 0.47 in this population.[12]
- Prospective validation of the use of the OAR in children 2–16 years old. For ankle fracture, the OAR had a Sn of 1.0 and a Sp of 0.24, while for midfoot fracture the Sn was 1.0 and the Sp was 0.36.[13]
- Prospective validation in an Asian population with twisting injuries. Results found the rule had a Sn of 0.9 and a Sp of 0.3, which they deemed to be not sensitive enough. When the investigators modified the rule to require radiographs for patients who could not bear weight *either* immediately after injury *or* in the ED (as opposed to *both* immediately after injury *and* in the ED), the Sn was found to be 0.99 and the use of the modified rule would have reduced foot and ankle radiographs by 28%.[14]
- Prospective validation of the OAR in a military population when used by a physical therapist and an orthopedic surgeon. For physical therapists the Sn was 1.0 and the Sp was 0.4 for ankle injuries. For foot injuries the Sn was 1.0 and the Sp was 0.79. For the orthopedic surgeon, the Sn was also 1.0 for both foot and ankle injuries, while the Sp was 0.79 and 0.46, respectively. Kappa coefficient for interobserver agreement between orthopedic surgeon and physical therapist was 0.82 for ankle injuries and 0.88 for foot injuries.[15]
- Prospective validation in Hong Kong EDs. For ankle injuries, the OAR had a Sn of 0.98 and a Sp of 0.41 and for midfoot injuries it had a Sn of 1.0 and a Sp of 0.44.[16]
- Prospective validation in Greek athletes and nonathletes. OAR was found to have a Sn of 1.0 for both ankle and midfoot fractures; Sp was 0.3 and 0.4 for ankle and midfoot fractures, respectively.[17]
- Prospective validation in ED of an urban teaching hospital in Australia. The Sn was found to be 1.0 for both ankle and midfoot fractures. The Sp was 0.16 for ankle fractures and 0.21 for midfoot fractures.[18]
- Prospective validation of the OAR by nurses found a Sn of 0.92 and a Sp of 0.36.[19]
- Prospective validation of the OAR when used by specialized ED nurses compared with junior doctors. For specialized ED nurses the Sn was 0.93 and the Sp was 0.49, whereas the Sn was 0.93 and Sp was 0.39 for the junior doctors, indicating the specially trained nurses could accurately implement the OAR.[20]
- Impact analysis of the implementation of the OAR by triage nurses before physician evaluation. Results indicated a statistically insignificant difference

in length of stay with the OAR group and there was no difference in patient satisfaction ratings.[21]

- Prospective validation of the OAR in Iran. Results indicated a Sn of 1.0 for both ankle and midfoot fractures; the Sp was 0.41 for malleolar fracture and 0.56 for midfoot fracture.[22]
- Attempted prospective validation for patients assessing themselves with the OAR. Results indicated poor interobserver agreement between patients and clinicians indicating that patients could not self-assess their injury using the OAR.[23]

## References

1. Stiell IG, Greenberg GH, McKnight RD, Nair RC, McDowell I, Worthington JR. A study to develop clinical decision rules for the use of radiography in acute ankle injuries. *Ann of Emerg Med*. 1992;21:384–390.

2. Stiell IG, Greenberg GH, McKnight RD, et al. Decision rules for the use of radiography in acute ankle injuries: refinement and prospective validation. *JAMA*. 1993;269:1127–1132.

3. Stiell IG, McKnight D, Greenberg GH, et al. Implementation of the Ottawa ankle rules. *JAMA*. 1994;271:827–832.

4. Pigman EC, Klug RK, Sanford S, Jolly BT. Evaluation of the Ottawa clinical decision rules for the use of radiography in acute ankle and midfoot injuries in the emergency department: an independent site assessment. *Ann Emerg Med*. 1994;24:41–45.

5. Kelly AM, Richards D, Kerr L, et al. Failed validation of a clinical decision rule for the use of radiography in acute ankle injury. *N Z Med J*. 1994;107:294–295.

6. Anis AH, Stiell IG, Stewart DG, Laupacis A. Cost-effectiveness analysis of the Ottawa ankle rules. *Ann Emerg Med*. 1995;26:422–428.

7. Lucchesi GM, Jackson RE, Peacock WF, Cerasani C, Swor RA. Sensitivity of the Ottawa rules. *Ann Emerg Med*. 1995;26:1–5.

8. Stiell I, Wells G, Laupacis A, et al. Multicentre trial to introduce the Ottawa ankle rules for use of radiography in acute ankle injuries. Multicentre Ankle Rule Study Group. *BMJ*. 1995;311:594–597.

9. Auleley GR, Ravaud P, Giraudeau B, et al. Implementation of the Ottawa ankle rules in France: a multicenter randomized controlled trial. *JAMA*. 1997;277:1935–1939.

10. Leddy JJ, Smolinski RJ, Lawrence J, Snyder JL, Priore RL. Prospective evaluation of the Ottawa Ankle rules in a university sports medicine center. With a modification to increase specificity for identifying malleolar fractures. *Am J Sports Med*. 1998;26:158–165.

11. Markert RJ, Walley ME, Guttman TG, Mehta R. A pooled analysis of the Ottawa ankle rules used on adults in the ED. *Am J Emerg Med*. 1998;16:564–567.

12. Libetta C, Burke D, Brennan P, Yassa J. Validation of the Ottawa ankle rules in children. *J Accid Emerg Med*. 1999;16:342–344.

13. Plint AC, Bulloch B, Osmond MH, et al. Validation of the Ottawa ankle rules in children with ankle injuries. *Acad Emerg Med*. 1999;6:1005–1009.

14. Tay SY, Thoo FL, Sitoh YY, Seow E, Wong HP. The Ottawa ankle rules in Asia: validating a clinical decision rule for requesting X-rays in twisting ankle and foot injuries. *J Emerg Med*. 1999;17:945–947.

15. Springer BA, Arciero RA, Tenuta JJ, Taylor DC. A prospective study of modified Ottawa ankle rules in a military population. *AM J Sports Med.* 2000;28:864–868.

16. Yuen MC, Sim SW, Lam HS, Tung WK. Validation of the Ottawa ankle rules in a Hong Kong ED. *Am J Emerg Med.* 2001;19:429–432.

17. Papacostas E, Malliaropoulos N, Papadopoulos A, Liouliakis C. Validation of Ottawa ankle rules protocol in Greek athletes: study in the emergency departments of a district general hospital and a sports injuries clinic. *Br J Sports Med.* 2001;35:445–447.

18. Broomhead A, Stuart P. Validation of the Ottawa ankle rules in Australia. *Emerg Med (Fremantle).* 2003;15:126–132.

19. Fiesseler F, Szucus P, Kec R, Richman PB. Can nurses appropriately interpret the Ottawa ankle rule? *Am J Emerg Med.* 2004;22:145–148.

20. Derksen RJ, Bakker FC, Geervliet PC, et al. Diagnostic accuracy and reproductility in the interpretation of Ottawa ankle and foot rules by specialized emergency nurses. *Am J Emerg Med.* 2005;23:725–729.

21. Fan J, Woolfrey K. The effect of triage-applied Ottawa ankle rules on the length of stay in a Canadian urgent care department: a randomized controlled trial. *Acad Emerg Med.* 2006;13:153–157.

22. Yazdani S, Jahandideh H, Ghofrani H. Validation of the Ottawa ankle rules in Iran: a prospective survey. *BMC Emerg Med.* 2006;6:3.

23. Blackham JE, Claridge T, Benger JR. Can patients apply the Ottawa ankle rules to themselves? *Emerg Med J.* 2008;25:750–751.

## FRACTURE

# Radiography of the Knee After Acute/Blunt Injury

## Ottawa Knee Rules[1]

### Predictor Variables

1. ≥ 55 years old
2. Tenderness at the head of the fibula
3. Isolated tenderness of the patella
4. Inability to flex the knee to 90°
5. Inability to bear weight both immediately *and* in the ED (four steps)

### Clinical Bottom Line

The Ottawa Knee Rules provide a sensitive set of predictor variables where if none are present, a knee fracture is unlikely and radiographs may not be needed. This rule has been validated as an effective screening tool; however, given the consequences of a missed knee fracture, it is recommended that clinicians consider the patient's status on this rule along with the full clinical picture when making decisions on whether to initiate treatment.

### Examination

- Tenderness at the head of the fibula (**Figure 4.5**)
  - Defined as tenderness at the proximal fibula

**Diagnostic**

**Level: I**

Knee Radiographs **Not** Indicated if:

**NONE** of the Predictor Variables Are Present

**Sensitivity 1.0** (95% CI 0.95–1.0) in All Cases

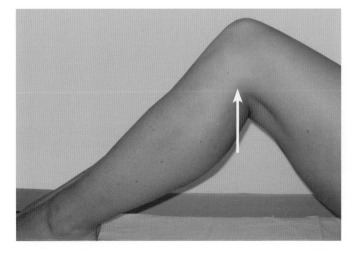

**Figure 4.5**
Palpation for tenderness at the head of the fibula.

- Isolated tenderness of the patella (**Figure 4.6**)
  - Defined as tenderness at the patella only, and no other areas of bone tenderness about the knee

**Figure 4.6**
Palpation for isolated tenderness of the patella.

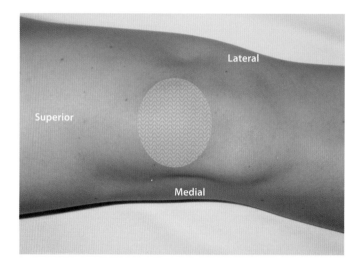

- Inability to flex the knee to 90° (**Figure 4.7**)
  - Measured with a goniometer: axis is aligned with the lateral femoral epicondyle; stationary arm is aligned with the femur pointing toward the greater trochanter; moving arm is aligned with the fibula pointing toward the lateral malleolus

**Figure 4.7**
Knee flexion range of motion.

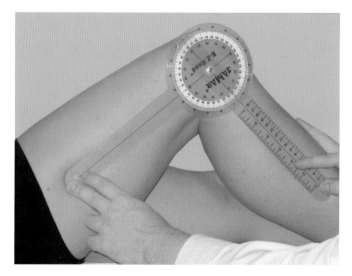

- Inability to bear weight both immediately and in the ED
  - Immediately after injury: examiner asks patient if he or she was able to bear weight for four steps immediately after the injury

■ Patient is instructed to walk for four steps (two foot contacts per side): if patient is unable due to pain, this variable is considered positive; if patient is able to bear weight on the affected limb with or without a limp, this variable is negative

## Study Specifics

### Inclusion Criteria

- Adult
- Acute blunt injuries of the knee regardless of mechanism of injury

### Exclusion Criteria

- Ages < 18
- Pregnant
- Isolated injuries of the skin without underlying soft-tissue or bone involvement
  - ■ Superficial lacerations
  - ■ Abrasions
  - ■ Puncture wounds
  - ■ Burns
- Referred from outside the hospital with radiographs
- Knee injury > 7 days previous
- Returning for reassessment of the same injury
- Altered level of consciousness
- Paraplegic
- Multiple trauma or other fractures

### Patient Characteristics

- N = 1047 subjects
- Mean age = 36 (+/− 25)
- Prevalence of clinically significant fractures = 6.3%
- Gender
  - ■ Female = 42%
  - ■ Male = 58%

### Definition of Positive (Reference Standard)

- Radiograph: presence or absence of any fracture of the knee or patella seen on standard plain knee radiography
  - ■ Knee was defined as the patella, head and neck of fibula, proximal 8 cm of tibia and distal 8 cm of femur

  - Clinically insignificant fractures were defined as any avulsion fragment that was < 5 mm in breadth and that was not associated with a complete tendon or ligament disruption
  - Radiographs were interpreted by independent radiologists who were blinded to the contents of the data-collection sheet
- Follow-up interview
  - Conducted because only 69% of patients received radiography in standard practice and the investigators could not demand that all patients undergo radiography for the purposes of the study
  - Patients who could not fulfill all of the following were recalled for reassessment and radiography
    - Pain feels better
    - Ability to walk is better
    - Does not require assistance to walk (crutches/cast/splint)
    - Has returned to usual occupational activities (work/household/school)
    - Has no plans to see a physician about knee injury

*Validation/Impact Analysis*

- Prospective validation. Results confirmed the application of the rule with a Sn of 1.0 (95% CI 0.94–1.0) and reliability ($\kappa$ value 0.77, 95% CI 0.65–0.89) between two physicians.[2]
- Prospective validation in an inner-city ED. Results confirmed the accuracy of the rule in an inner-city population with a Sn of 0.98 (95% CI 0.88–0.99) and a negative LR of 0.12 (95% CI 0.02–0.60).[3]
- Prospective validation in 11 emergency departments. Results confirmed the application of the rule with a Sn of 1.0 (95% CI 0.96–1.0) and found a potential 49% reduction in the use of radiography.[4]
- Prospective validation of the use of the rule by medical students and surgery residents. Results indicated a Sn of 1.0 and a 25% reduction in radiography requests.[5]
- Prospective multicenter validation for the use of the rule in children. Results indicated a Sn of 1.0 (95% CI 0.95–1.0) and a 31.2% reduction in radiography.[6]
- Prospective validation of the rule by junior doctors in the United Kingdom. Results indicated a Sn of 1.0 (95% CI 0.72–1.0), but a nonsignificant decrease in the use of radiography.[7]
- Prospective validation of the rule. Results indicated a Sn of 1.0 and a reduction in radiographs by 35%.[8]

## References

1. Stiell IG, Greenberg GH, Wells GA, et al. Derivation of a decision rule for the use of radiography in acute knee injuries. *Ann Emerg Med*. 1995;26:405–413.

2. Stiell IG, Greenberg GH, Wells GA, et al. Prospective validation of a decision rule for the use of radiography in acute knee injuries. *JAMA*. 1996;275:641–642.

3. Tigges S, Pitts S, Mukundan S, Morrison D, Olson M, Shahriara A. External validation of the Ottawa knee rules in an urban trauma center in the United States. *Am J Roentgenol*. 1999;172:1069–1071.

4. Emparanza JI, Aginaga JR. Validation of the Ottawa knee rules. *Ann Emerg Med*. 2000;38:364–368.

5. Ketelslegers E, Collard X, Vande Berg B, et al. Validation of the Ottawa knee rules in an emergency teaching centre. *Eur Radiol*. 2002;12:1218–1220.

6. Bulloch B, Neto G, Plint A, et al. Validation of the Ottawa knee rule in children: a multicenter study. *Ann Emerg Med*. 2003;42:48–55.

7. Atkinson P, Boyle A, Chisholm E. X-ray requesting patterns before and after introduction of the Ottawa knee rules in a UK emergency department. *Eur J Emerg Med*. 2004;11:204–207.

8. Jenny JY, Boeri C, El Amrani H, et al. Should plain X-rays be routinely performed after blunt knee trauma? A prospective analysis. *J Trauma*. 2005;58:1179–1182.

## FRACTURE

# Radiography of the Knee After Acute/Blunt Injury

## Pittsburgh Knee Rules[1]

| **Diagnostic** |
| :--- |

| **Level: II** |
| :--- |

Knee Radiographs
**Not** Indicated if:

**NO** Fall or Blunt
Trauma Mechanisms of
Injury

**Sensitivity 0.9**

### Predictor Variables

**1.** Fall or blunt trauma mechanism of injury

*and*

- Inability to ambulate initially or in the emergency department (four steps)

*or*

- Age (younger than 12 or older than 50)

### Clinical Bottom Line

The Pittsburgh Knee Rules provide a sensitive set of predictor variables to determine whether an individual requires plain films to rule out a knee fracture after an acute/blunt injury. The addition of "inability to ambulate" and "age" serve to increase specificity, but they do not influence the sensitivity of the test. This rule has been validated as an effective screening tool; however, given the consequences of a missed knee fracture, it is recommended that clinicians consider the patient's status on this rule along with the full clinical picture when making decisions on whether to initiate treatment.

### Study Specifics

*Inclusion Criteria*

- All patients presenting with acute knee injuries

*Exclusion Criteria*

- Injuries > 1 week old
- Isolated skin injuries (superficial lacerations or abrasions)
- Had prior knee surgery
- Returning for reassessment of the same knee injury

*Patient Characteristics*

- N = 201 subjects
- Gender

- ▪ Female = 47%
- ▪ Male = 53%
- Prevalence of clinically significant fractures = 6%

*Definition of Positive (Reference Standard)*

- Presence of any knee fracture, as detected on radiographs

*Validation*

- Prospective validation performed in the same sample of patients. Results indicated a Sn of 1.0 (95% CI 0.74–1.0) and a Sp of 0.79 (95% CI 0.70–0.85).[1]
- Prospective validation indicated the Pittsburgh rule possesses a Sp of 0.60 (95% CI 0.56–0.64) and a Sn of 0.99 (95% CI 0.94–1.0) compared to the Ottawa Knee Rules, which had a Sn of 0.97 (95% CI 0.90–0.99) and a Sp of 0.27 (95% CI 0.23–0.30).[2]

## References

1. Seaberg DC, Jackson R. Clinical decision rule for knee radiographs. *Am J Emerg Med.* 1994;12:541–543.
2. Seaberg DC, Yealy DM, Lukens T, Auble T, Mathias S. Multicenter comparison of two clinical decision rules for the use of radiography in acute, high-risk knee injuries. *Ann Emerg Med.* 1998;32:8–13.

## FRACTURE

# Indications for Cervical Spine Radiography

## Canadian Cervical Spine Rules[1]

**Diagnostic**

**Level: II**

If Decision-Making Algorithm Leads to "No Radiography"

For **No** Fracture Present

**Sensitivity 1.0** (95% CI 0.98–1.0)

### Predictor Variables

Any *high-risk factors* would necessitate *radiographs:*
- Age ≥ 65
- Dangerous mechanism of injury [a]
- Paresthesias in extremities

*If No:* Any low-risk factors that would allow for safe assessment of ROM:
- Simple rear-end MVC [b]
- Sitting position in the ED
- Ambulatory at any time
- Delayed onset of neck pain (not immediate)
- Absence of mid-cervical tenderness

*If Yes:* Active neck rotation is ≥ 45° bilaterally (regardless of pain): *Radiographs are not needed.*

*If No:* No low-risk factors present or the patient is unable to rotate the neck ≥ 45° in both directions: *Radiographs should be requested.*[a,b]

### Clinical Bottom Line

The Canadian Cervical Spine Rules provide a sensitive cluster of signs and symptoms, and if they lead to "No Radiography," then radiograph to rule out cervical spine fracture is likely not indicated. This rule has been validated as an effective screening tool; however, given the consequences of a missed cervical spine fracture, it is recommended that clinicians consider the patient's status on this rule along with the full clinical picture when making decisions on whether to initiate treatment.

---

a  Dangerous mechanism includes: fall from ≥1 meter/five stairs, axial load to head (i.e., diving), MVC high speed (> 100 km/hr, rollover, ejection), motorized recreational vehicles, bicycle collision

b  Simple rear-end MVC excludes: pushed into oncoming traffic, hit by bus/large truck, rollover, hit by high-speed vehicle

## Study Specifics

### Inclusion Criteria

- Consecutive adult patients presenting to the ED after acute blunt trauma to the head or neck
- Neck pain from any mechanism of injury
- No neck pain but had some visible injury above the clavicles, had not been ambulatory, and had sustained a dangerous mechanism of injury
- Glasgow Coma Scale (GCS) of 15
- Stable vital signs
  - Systolic blood pressure greater than 90 mmHg
  - Respiratory rate between 10 and 24 breaths per minute

### Exclusion Criteria

- < 16 years old
- Only minor injuries, such as simple lacerations, and did not fulfill the first two inclusion criteria above
- GCS score < 15
- Grossly abnormal vital signs
- Injured > 48 hours previously
- Penetrating trauma
- Presented with acute paralysis
- Known vertebral disease (ankylosing spondylitis, rheumatoid arthritis, spinal stenosis, or previous cervical surgery)
- Had returned for reassessment of the same injury
- Pregnancy
- Subjects without radiography who could not be contacted on 14 day follow-up

### Patient Characteristics

- N = 8924 subjects
- Mean age = 36.7 (+/− 16)
- Prevalence of clinically significant cervical spine injury = 1.7%
- Gender
  - Female = 48%
  - Male = 52%

*Definition of Positive (Reference Standard)*

- Clinically important cervical spine injury
  - Defined as any fracture, dislocation, or ligamentous instability demonstrated by diagnostic imaging

*Definition of Negative*

- Clinically unimportant cervical spine injury was not considered positive
  - Patient neurologically intact with any of the following injuries
    - Isolated avulsion fracture of an osteophyte
    - Isolated fracture of a transverse process not involving a facet joint
    - Isolated fracture of a spinous process not involving the lamina
    - Simple compression fracture involving < 25% of the vertebral body height

*Validation*

- Prospective validation study comparing the Canadian Cervical Spine Rules with unstructured physician judgment. Results indicate the Canadian rule is more Sn (1.0) and Sp (0.54) compared to unstructured judgment (Sn 0.92 and Sp 0.44).[2]
- Prospective validation study comparing the Canadian Cervical Spine Rules with NEXUS. Results indicate the Canadian rule is more Sn (0.99) and Sp (0.45) compared to NEXUS II (Sn 0.91 and Sp 0.37).[3]

## References

1. Stiell IG, Wells GA, Vandemheen KL, et al. The Canadian C-spine rule for radiography in alert and stable trauma patients. *JAMA*. 2001;286:1841–1848.
2. Bandiera G, Stiell IG, Wells GA, et al. The Canadian C-spine rule performs better than unstructured physician judgment. *Ann Emerg Med*. 2003;42:395–402.
3. Stiell IG, Clement CM, McKnight RD, et al. The Canadian C-spine rule versus the NEXUS low-risk criteria in patients with trauma. *NEJM*. 2003;349:2510–2518.

## HEAD INJURY

# Indications for Computed Tomography (CT) Scan After Head Injury

## NEXUS II[1]

### Predictor Variables

1. Evidence of significant skull fracture
2. Scalp hematoma
3. Neurologic deficit
4. Altered level of alertness
5. Abnormal behavior
6. Coagulopathy
7. Persistent vomiting
8. Age ≥ 65 years old

### Clinical Bottom Line

NEXUS II provides a sensitive set of predictor variables to determine whether an individual requires a CT scan after blunt head injury to rule out clinically important brain injury. This rule has been validated as an effective screening tool; however, given the consequences of a missed head injury, it is recommended that clinicians consider the patient's status on this rule along with the full clinical picture when making decisions on whether to initiate treatment.

### Examination

- Evidence of significant skull fracture
  - Includes, but is not limited to, any signs of basilar skull fracture, signs of depressed or diastatic skull fracture
- Neurologic deficit
  - Present if a patient exhibits any of the following: abnormal Glasgow Coma Scale score, motor deficit, gait abnormality, abnormal cerebellar function, or cranial nerve abnormality
- Altered level of alertness
  - Evidenced by a variety of findings, including but not limited to a Glasgow Coma Scale score of 14 or less; delayed or inappropriate response to external stimuli; excessive somnolence; disorientation to

**Diagnostic**

**Level: II**

CT Scan **Not** Indicated if:

**NO** Predictor Variables Present

**Sensitivity 0.98** (95% CI 0.97–0.99) in All Cases

**Sensitivity 0.95** (95% CI 0.92–0.97) in Those with GCS of 15

person, place, time, or events; inability to remember three objects at 5 minutes; perseverating speech; and other findings

- Abnormal behavior
  - Any inappropriate action displayed by the victim. It includes such things as excessive agitation, inconsolability, refusal to cooperate, lack of affective response to questions or events, and violent activity
- Coagulopathy
  - Any impairment of normal blood clotting such as occurs in hemophilia, secondary to medications (e.g., coumadin, heparin, aspirin), in hepatic insufficiency, and in other conditions

## Study Specifics

### Inclusion Criteria

- Blunt head trauma patients for whom CT scan was ordered

### Exclusion Criteria

- Penetrating trauma
- Infections
- Cerebrovascular accidents
- Tumors
- Other atraumatic indications for CT

### Patient Characteristics

- N = 13,728 subjects
- Median age = 37
- Prevalence of clinically important intracranial injuries = 6.7%
- Gender
  - Female = 34%
  - Male = 66%

### Definition of Positive (Reference Standard)

- Any injury that may require surgical intervention, or lead to rapid deterioration, or long-term injury, as diagnosed by CT
  - Mass effect or sulcal effacement
  - Signs of herniation
  - Basal cistern compression or midline shift
  - Substantial epidural or subdural hematomas (greater than 1.0 cm in width, or causing mass effect)

- Extensive subarachnoid hemorrhage
- Hemorrhage in the posterior fossa
- Intraventricular hemorrhage
- Bilateral hemorrhage of any type
- Depressed or diastatic skull fracture
- Pneumocephalus
- Diffuse cerebral edema
- Diffuse axonal injury

### Validation

- Validated in children 0–18 years with similarly high sensitivity (published as abstract only; sensitivity not reported).[2]
- External validation of several CDRs for CT scan in head injury patients. The NEXUS II and Scandinavian clinical decision aids had the best combination of Sn and Sp. NEXUS II Sn was 1.0 (95% CI 0.96–1.0) with a Sp of 0.44 (95% CI 0.43–0.46) for injuries that would require surgical intervention, and it had a Sn of 0.97 (95% CI 0.96–0.98) and a Sp of 0.47 (95% CI 0.46–0.48) for any lesion.[3]

## References

1. Mower WR, Hoffman JR, Herbert M, Wolfson AB, Pollack CV Jr, Zucker MI. Developing a decision instrument to guide computed tomographic imaging of blunt head injury patients. *J Trauma*. 2005;59:954–959.
2. Oman JA, Cooper RJ, Holmes JF, et al. Performance of a decision rule to predict need for computed tomography among children with blunt head trauma. *Pediatrics*. 2006;117:e238–e246.
3. Stein SC, Fabbri A, Servandei F, Glick HA. A critical comparison of clinical decision instruments for computed tomographic scanning in mild closed traumatic brain injury in adolescents and adults. *Ann Emerg Med*. 2009;53:180–188.

HEAD INJURY

# Computed Tomography (CT) in Patients with Minor Head Injury[1]

## Computed Tomography Head Rules

| Diagnostic |
| --- |
| **Level: II** |
| Patient is **Not** a High Risk for Neurological Intervention if: |
| **NO** Predictor Variables Present |
| **Sensitivity 1.0** (95% CI 0.9–1.0) |
| Patient is **Not** a High Risk for Clinically Important Brain Injury if: |
| **No** Predictor Variables Present |
| **Sensitivity 0.98** (95% CI 0.96–0.99) |

### Predictor Variables

- High risk (neurological intervention)
  1. Glascow Coma Scale (GCS) < 15 at 2 hours after injury
  2. Suspected open or depressed skull fracture
  3. Any sign of basal skull fracture (hemotympanum, "raccoon" eyes, cerebrospinal fluid otorrhea/rhinorrhea, Battle's sign)
  4. Vomiting ≥ 2 episodes
  5. Age ≥ 65 years
- Medium risk (brain injury on CT)
  1. Amnesia before impact > 30 minutes
  2. Dangerous mechanism
     - Pedestrian struck by motor vehicle, occupant ejected from motor vehicle, fall from height > 3 feet or 5 stairs

### Clinical Bottom Line

The Canadian CT head rules provide a sensitive set of predictor variables to determine whether an individual requires a CT scan after blunt head injury to rule out clinically important brain injury (medium risk) or neurological intervention (high risk). Validation studies indicate that it is more specific than the New Orleans Criteria (NOC), and therefore has greater potential to decrease CT scan use; however, it is less sensitive in identifying any lesions on CT. Despite validation, given the consequences of a missed head injury, it is recommended that clinicians consider the patient's entire clinical picture in addition to this CPR.

### Study Specifics

*Inclusion Criteria*

- Patients presenting to ED after sustaining acute minor head injury
- All of the following
  - Blunt trauma to the head resulting in witnessed loss of consciousness, definite amnesia, or witnessed disorientation

  ▪ Initial emergency department GCS score of ≥ 13 as determined by the treating physician
  ▪ Injury within the past 24 hours

## Exclusion Criteria

- Ages < 16
- Minimal head injury
  ▪ No loss of consciousness, amnesia, or disorientation
- No clear history of trauma as the primary event
- Obvious penetrating skull injury or obvious depressed fracture
- Acute focal neurological deficit
- Unstable vital signs associated with major trauma
- Seizure before assessment in the ED
- Bleeding disorder or used oral anticoagulants (i.e., Coumadin)
- Had returned for reassessment of the same head injury
- Pregnancy
- Was not able to be contacted for 14-day questionnaire if no CT scan was initially performed

## Patient Characteristics

- N = 3121 subjects
- Mean age = 38.7 (+/– 18)
- Percentage of subjects requiring neurological intervention = 1%
- Prevalence of clinically important head injury on CT scan = 8%
- Gender
  ▪ Female = 41%
  ▪ Male = 69%

## Definition of Positive (Reference Standard)

- Need for neurological intervention, defined as
  ▪ Death within 7 days secondary to head injury
  ▪ The need for any of the following procedures within 7 days
    • Craniotomy
    • Elevation of skull fracture
    • Intracranial pressure monitoring
    • Intubation for head injury shown on CT scan
- Clinically important brain injury on CT scan defined as
  ▪ Any acute brain finding revealed on CT and which would normally require admission to hospital and neurological follow-up

- Clinically unimportant brain injuries included any of the following in neurologically intact subjects
  - Solitary contusion less than 5 mm in diameter
  - Localized subarachnoid blood less than 1 mm thick
  - Isolated pneumocephaly or closed, depressed skull fracture not through the inner table
- Subjects who did not undergo head CT were contacted within 14 days for a phone interview and were classified as not having a clinically important brain injury if they met all of the following. Those who did not meet all of the following were recalled for clinical reassessment and CT
  - Headache absent or mild
  - No complaints of memory or concentration problems
  - No seizure of focal motor findings
  - Weighted error score of no more than 10 out of 28 on the Katzman Short Orientation–Memory–Concentration Test
  - Had returned to normal daily activities (work, housework, or school)

*Validation/Impact Analysis*

- Prospective validation comparing the Canadian CT Head Rule (CCHR) with the NOC. Results found that for identifying lesions requiring neurosurgical intervention, CCHR had a Sn of 1.0 (95% CI 0.6–1.0) and a Sp of 0.76 (95% CI 0.74–0.78), and for clinically important brain injury it had a Sn of 1.0 (95% CI 0.96–1.0) and a Sp of 0.51 (95% CI 0.48–0.53).[2]
- Prospective external validation comparing the CCHR with the NOC in a broader population than either was derived in. Results found that for lesions requiring neurosurgical intervention, CCHR had a Sn of 1.0 (95% CI 0.65–1.0) and a Sp of .37 (95% CI 0.34–0.41), and for "Important CT findings" it had a Sn of 0.84 (95% CI 0.78–0.89) and a Sp of 0.39 (95% CI 0.36–0.42). Additionally, use of the rule would have led to a 37% reduction in the use of CT scans.[3]
- Retrospective validation of several decision rules for CT scans in minor head injury. Results found that for a lesion requiring surgery CCHR had a Sn of 0.99 (95% CI 0.94–1.0) and a Sp of 0.45 (95% CI 0.44–0.46), and for any lesion, it had a Sn of 0.99 (95% CI 0.98–1.0) and a Sp of 0.47 (0.46–0.48).[4]

## References

1. Stiell IG, Wells GA, Vandemheen K, et al. The Canadian CT Head Rule for patients with minor head injury. *Lancet*. 2001;357:1391–1396.
2. Stiell IG, Clement CM, Rowe BH, et al. Comparison of the Canadian CT Head Rule and the New Orleans Criteria in patients with minor head injury. *JAMA*. 2005;294:1511–1518.

3. Smits M, Dippel DW, de Haan GG, et al. External validation of the Canadian CT Head Rule and the New Orleans Criteria for CT scanning in patients with minor head injury. *JAMA*. 2005;294:1519–1525.
4. Stein SC, Fabbri A, Servadei F, Glick HA. A critical comparison of clinical decision instruments for computed tomographic scanning in mild closed traumatic brain injury in adolescents and adults. *Ann Emerg Med*. 2009;53:180–188.

HEAD INJURY

# Computed Tomography (CT) in Patients with Minor Head Injury

## New Orleans Criteria (NOC)[1]

**Diagnostic**

**Level: II**

CT Scan **Not** Indicated if:

**NO** Predictor Variables Present

**Sensitivity 1.0**
(95% CI 0.95–1.0)

### Predictor Variables

1. Headache
   - Defined as any head pain
2. Vomiting
   - Defined as any emesis after the traumatic event
3. Age > 60 years old
4. Drug or alcohol intoxication
   - As determined on the basis of the history obtained from the patient or a witness and suggestive findings on physical exam such as slurred speech or the odor of alcohol on the breath
5. Deficits in short-term memory
   - Defined as persistent anterograde amnesia in a patient with an otherwise normal score on the GCS
6. Physical evidence of trauma above the clavicles
   - Defined as any external evidence of injury including contusions, abrasions, lacerations, deformities, and signs of facial or skull fracture
7. Seizure
   - Defined as a suspected or witnessed seizure after the traumatic event

### Clinical Bottom Line

The NOC provides a set of predictor variables to determine whether an individual requires a computed tomography (CT) scan to rule out significant intracranial injury after acute/blunt head trauma. This rule has been validated as an effective screening tool; however, given the consequences of a missed head injury, it is recommended that clinicians consider the patient's status on this rule along with the full clinical picture when making decisions on whether to initiate treatment.

## Study Specifics

*Inclusion Criteria*

- Ages ≥ 3
- Presented to the emergency department within 24 hours of injury
- Minor head injury was defined as loss of consciousness in patients with normal findings on a brief neurologic examination (normal cranial nerves and normal strength and sensation in the arms and legs) and a score of 15 on the GCS, as determined by a physician on the patient's arrival at the ED
  - Loss of consciousness was confirmed if a witness or the patient reported loss of consciousness by the patient or if the patient could not remember the traumatic event

*Exclusion Criteria*

- Patients who declined CT scanning
- Concurrent injuries that precluded the use of CT scanning
- Reported no loss of consciousness or amnesia

*Patient Characteristics*

- N = 520 subjects
- Mean age = 36
- Gender
  - Female = 35%
  - Male = 65%
- Prevalence of positive CT scans = 6.9%

*Definition of Positive (Reference Standard)*

- Presence of an acute traumatic intracranial lesion on a CT scan
  - Subdural, epidural, or parenchymal hematoma
  - Subarachnoid hemorrhage
  - Cerebral contusion
  - Depressed skull fracture

*Validation/Impact Analysis*

- Phase 2 of the derivation study prospectively validated the NOC with 909 consecutive patients. Results indicated the rule had a Sn of 1.0 (95% CI 0.95–1.0) and a Sp of 0.25 (95% CI 0.22–0.28).[1]

- Prospective validation in children 5–17 years old. Results indicated a Sn of 1.0 (95% CI 0.73–1.0), and Sp ranged from 0.24 to 0.3. CT scans could have safely been reduced by 23% using the decision rule.[2]
- Prospective external validation comparing the CCHR with the NOC. Results found that for identifying lesions requiring neurosurgical intervention, the NOC had a Sn of 1.0 (95% CI 0.63–1.0) and a Sp of 0.12 (95% CI 0.11–0.14), and for any clinically important brain injury, NOC had a Sn of 1.0 (95% CI 0.96–1.0) and a Sp of 0.13 (95% CI 0.11–0.14).[3]
- External, prospective validation comparing the NOC with the CCHR. Results found that for identifying lesions requiring neurosurgical intervention, the NOC had a Sn of 1.0 (95% CI 0.34–1.0) and a Sp of 0.05 (0.03–0.08), and for "Important CT finding," it had a Sn of 0.98 (95% CI 0.92–0.99) and a Sp of 0.06 (95% CI 0.03–0.09). Additionally, it would have reduced the use of CT scans by 5%.[4]
- Retrospective external validation comparing several clinical decision instruments. Results found that for surgical lesions, the NOC had a Sn of 0.99 (95% CI 0.94–1.0) and a Sp of 0.31 (95% CI 0.32–0.34), and for any lesion the NOC had a Sn of 0.99 (95% CI 0.98–1.0) and a Sp of 0.33 (95% CI 0.32–0.34).[5]

## References

1. Haydel MJ, Preston CA, Mills TJ, Luber S, Blaudeau E, DeBlieus PM. Indications for computed tomography in patients with minor head injury. *NEJM*. 2000;242:100–106.
2. Haydel MJ, Shembekar AD. Prediction of intracranial injury in children aged five years and older with loss of consciousness after minor head injury due to nontrivial mechanisms. *Ann Emerg Med*. 2003;42(4):507–514.
3. Stiell IG, Clement CM, Rowe BH, et al. Comparison of the Canadian CT Head Rule and the New Orleans Criteria in patients with minor head injury. *JAMA*. 2005;294:1511–1518.
4. Smits M, Dippel DW, de Haan GG, et al. External validation of the Canadian CT Head Rule and the New Orleans Criteria for CT scanning in patients with minor head injury. *JAMA*. 2005;294:1519–1525.
5. Stein SC, Fabbri A, Servadei F, Glick HA. A critical comparison of clinical decision instruments for computed tomographic scanning in mild closed traumatic brain injury in adolescents and adults. *Ann Emerg Med*. 2009;53:180–188.

OSTEOPOROSIS

# Bone Densitometry in Women

## The Osteoporosis Risk Assessment Instrument (ORAI)[1]

### Predictor Variables

| Variable | Score |
|---|---|
| **1.** Age | |
| **a.** ≥ 75 | 15 |
| **b.** 65–74 | 9 |
| **c.** 55–64 | 5 |
| **d.** 45–54 | 0 |
| **2.** Weight in kg | |
| **a.** < 60 | 9 |
| **b.** 60–69 | 3 |
| **c.** ≥ 70 | 0 |
| **3.** Current Estrogen Use | |
| **a.** No | 2 |
| **b.** Yes | 0 |

**Diagnostic**

**Level: II**

Bone Densitometry
**Not** Indicated if:

Score Is ≤ **8**

**Sensitivity 0.9**
(95% CI 0.8–0.9)

### Clinical Bottom Line

The Osteoporosis Risk Assessment Instrument (ORAI) can be used with relative confidence to exclude patients who do not need bone densitometry due to low bone mineral density (BMD). Due to the low specificity and the high number of false positives, the tool cannot reliably identify patients for whom testing is indicated. This rule has been validated and may be applied to practice within the confines of the study's parameters.

### Study Specifics

*Inclusion Criteria*

- Noninstitutionalized
- ≥ 45 years old
- Women
- Mini-Mental State Score > 20
- Had undergone dual-energy X-ray absorptiometry (DXA) testing at the femoral neck and lumbar spine

- Reside within 50 km of study center
- Fluent in English, French, or Chinese

*Exclusion Criteria*

- Diagnosis of osteoporosis
- Taking bone-active medications other than ovarian hormones (calcitonin, biphosphonates, fluoride)
- Native populations residing in the northern regions of the country (Canada)

*Patient Characteristics*

- N = 926 subjects
- Mean age (y) = 62.8 (+/− 9.36)
- Prevalence of low BMD = 23%
- Race = 95% white, 3% Asian

*Definition of Positive (Reference Standard)*

- Low BMD, diagnosed by bone densitometry, was defined as a T score of ≥ 2.0 standard deviations below the mean BMD in young Canadian women at the femoral neck or lumbar spine.

*Validation*

- Retrospective, internal validation arm of the original derivation study. Results indicated a Sn of 0.93 (95% CI 0.86–0.97) and a Sp of 0.46 (95% CI 0.41–0.51%).[1]
- Retrospective, external validation of 2365 Canadian postmenopausal women. Results indicated a Sn of 0.94 (95% CI 0.92–0.96) and a Sp of 0.56 (95% CI 0.53–0.69) to identify women with a BMD T score of < −2.0.[2]
- Retrospective, external validation of 4035 Caucasian, Belgian, postmenopausal women. Results indicated an overall Sn of 0.90 and a Sp of 0.42 to identify women with a BMD T score of ≤ −2.5 at three sites (total hip, femoral neck, and L2–L4 spine). The cutoff score was ≥ 8.[3]
- Retrospective, external validation of 202 postmenopausal women residing in Minnesota. Results indicated a Sn of 0.98 (95% CI 0.51–1.0) and a Sp of 0.40 (95 CI 0.30–0.56) to identify women with a BMD T score of ≤ −2.5 at the femoral neck.[4]
- Retrospective, external validation of 2539 postmenopausal women in Belgium. Threshold score on the ORAI was ≥ 8. Results indicated a Sn of 0.89 (95% CI 0.82–0.93) and a Sp of 0.46 (95% CI 0.44–0.48) to identify women with a BMD T score of ≤ −2.5 at the femoral neck.[5]

- Retrospective, external validation of 2016 Danish perimenopausal and early postmenopausal women. Results indicated a Sn of 0.50 (95% CI 0.44–0.56) and a Sp of 0.75 (95% CI 0.73–0.77) to identify women with a BMD T score of ≤ 2.0 at the femoral neck.[6]
- Retrospective, external validation of 665 Spanish postmenopausal women. Results indicated a Sn of 0.64 (95% CI 0.55–0.73) and a Sp of 0.59 (95% CI 0.55–0.63) to identify women with a BMD T score of ≤ –2.5 at the lumbar spine or femoral neck.[7]
- Retrospective, external validation of 1127 Japanese postmenopausal women. Results indicated a Sn of 0.89 and a Sp of 0.39 to identify women with a spinal BMD T score of ≤ –2.5 with a cutoff score of ≥ 15.[8]
- Retrospective, external validation of 1102 postmenopausal women from the United States. Results indicated a Sn of 0.90 (95% CI 0.85–0.95) and a Sp of 0.52 (95% CI 0.49–0.55) to identify women with BMD T scores ≤ –2.5 measured at the femoral neck.[9]

## References

1. Cadarette SM, Jaglal SB, Kreiger N, McIsaac WJ, Darlington GA, Tu JV. Development and validation of the osteoporosis risk assessment instrument to facilitate selection of women for bone densitometry. *CMAJ*. 2000;162:1289–1294.
2. Cadarette SM, Jaglal SB, Murray TM, McIsaac WJ, Joseph L, Brown JP. Evaluation of decision rules for referring women for bone densitometry by duel-energy X-ray absorptiometry. *JAMA*. 2001;286:57–63.
3. Richy F, Gourlay M, Ross PD, et al. Validation and comparative evaluation of the osteoporosis self-assessment tool in a Caucasian population from Belgium. *QJM*. 2004;97:39–46.
4. Mauck KF, Cuddihy MT, Atkinson EJ, Melton LJ III. Use of clinical prediction rules in detecting osteoporosis in a population-based sample of postmenopausal women. *Arch Intern Med*. 2005;165:530–536.
5. Gourlay ML, Miller WC, Richy F, Garrett JM, Hanson LC, Reginster JY. Performance of osteoporosis risk assessment tools in postmenopausal women aged 45–64 years. *Osteoporosis Int*. 2005;16:921–927.
6. Rud B, Jensen JEB, Mosekilde L, Nielsen SP, Hilden J, Abrahamsen B. Performance of four clinical screening tools to select peri- and early postmenopausal women for dual X-ray absorptiometry. *Osteopros Int*. 2005;16:764–772.
7. Martinez-Aguila D, Gomez-Vaquero C, Rozadilla A, Romera M, Narvaez J, Nolla JM. Decision rules for selecting women for bone mineral density testing: application in postmenopausal women referred to a bone densitometry unit. *J Rheumatol*. 2007;34:1307–1312.
8. Fujiwara S, Masunari N, Suzuki G, Ross PD. Performance of osteoporosis risk indices in a Japanese population. *Ther Res Clin Exp*. 2001;62:586–594.
9. Geusens P, Hochberg MC, van der Voort DJ, et al. Performance of risk indices for identifying low bone mineral density in postmenopausal women. *Mayo Clinic Proceedings*. 2002;77:629–637.

OSTEOPOROSIS

# Bone Densitometry in Women

## Simple Calculated Osteoporosis Risk Estimation (SCORE)[1]

**Diagnostic**

**Level: II**

Bone Densitometry **Not** Indicated if:

Score Is ≤ **5**

**Sensitivity 0.9**
(95% CI 0.8–0.9)

### Predictor Variables

| Variable | Score | If Woman |
|---|---|---|
| **1.** Race | 5 | is *not* black |
| **2.** Rheumatoid arthritis | 4 | *has* rheumatoid arthritis |
| **3.** History of fractures | 4 | adds score for *each type* (wrist, rib, hip) of nontraumatic fracture after age 45 (max score = 12) |
| **4.** Age | 3 | multiplies by first digit of age in years (i.e., 54 years old is 5 × 3 or 15 points) |
| **5.** Estrogen | 1 | has *never* received estrogen therapy |
| **6.** Weight | −1 | multiplies weight divided by 10 and truncated to integer (i.e., 130 pounds would be −1 × 13 or −13) |

### Example of the Scoring System

A 59-year-old, 160-pound white woman with no history of fractures or Rheumatoid Arthritis (RA), and has never received estrogen therapy: 5 points for race, 0 points for RA, 4 × 0 = 0 points for fracture, 5 × 3 = 15 points for age, 1 point for not receiving estrogen therapy, −1 × 16 = −6 points for weight. Total = 5 + 0 + 0 + 15 + 1 − 16 = 5 points. Threshold score is ≤ 5; hence a referral for bone densitometry study is not necessary.

### Clinical Bottom Line

This CPR is a sensitive cluster of items, and individuals with ≤ 5 points can be excluded from requiring bone densitometry testing. Due to the low specificity and high numbers of false positives, the tool cannot reliably identify individuals for whom testing is indicated. This rule has been validated and may be applied to practice within the confines of the study's parameters.

## Study Specifics

*Inclusion Criteria*

- Ages ≥ 45
- Female
- Community dwelling
- Postmenopausal (amenorrheic for at least 6 months)
- Able to read English and provide informed consent

*Exclusion Criteria*

- Significant scoliosis, trauma, or sequelae or orthopedic procedures prohibiting bone mineral density (BMD) measurements of the spine or hip using X-ray absorptiometry
- Metabolic bone disease (other than osteoporosis)
- Cancer with metastasis to bone
- Renal impairment (serum creatinine > 2.5mg/dL)

*Patient Characteristics*

- N = 1279 subjects
- Mean age = 61.5 (+/− 9.6)
- Prevalence of low BMD = 38%
- Race = 89% white, 6% black, 3% Hispanic

*Definition of Positive (Reference Standard)*

- Low BMD, diagnosed by bone densitometry, was defined as a T score at the femoral neck of ≥ 2 standard deviations below the mean BMD in young, healthy white women

*Validation*

- Prospective, internal validation of postmenopausal, community-dwelling women seen in outpatient practices. Results indicated a Sn of 0.91 (95% CI 0.81–0.96) and a Sp of 0.40 (95% CI 0.30–0.52) to detect a BMD T score of ≤ −2.0 at the femoral neck. Excellent reliability of the questionnaire noted with an ICC of 0.96.[1]
- Retrospective validation of postmenopausal Canadian women. Results indicated a Sn of 0.91 (95% CI 0.86–.94) and a Sp of 0.32 (95% CI 0.25–0.39) to detect a BMD T score of ≤ −2.0 at either the femoral neck or lumbar spine.[2]

- Retrospective validation of postmenopausal Canadian women. Results indicated a Sn of 0.98 (95% CI 0.96–0.99) and a Sp of 0.69 (95% CI 0.66–0.73) to identify women with a BMD T score of < –2.0 at the femoral neck.[3]
- Retrospective validation of postmenopausal Belgian women. Results indicated a Sn of 0.92 and a Sp of 0.27 to identify women with a BMD T score of ≤ –2.5 at the femoral neck, total hip, and L2–L4 spine.[4]
- Retrospective validation of postmenopausal Belgian women. Results indicated an overall Sn of 0.97 and a Sp of 0.33 to identify women with a BMD T score of ≤ –2.5 at three sites (total hip, femoral neck, and L2–L4 spine). The cutoff score used was ≥ 7.[5]
- Retrospective validation of postmenopausal women who reside in Minnesota. Results indicated a Sn of 1.0 (95% CI 0.55–1.0) and a Sp of 0.29 (95% CI 0.18–0.48) to detect a BMD T score of ≤ –2.5 at the femoral neck.[6]
- Retrospective validation of postmenopausal Belgian women. Threshold score on SCORE was ≥ 7. Sn was 0.89 (95% CI 0.82–0.93) and Sp was 0.40 (95% CI 0.38–0.42) to identify women with a BMD T score of ≤ –2.5 at the femoral neck.[7]
- Retrospective validation of perimenopausal and early postmenopausal Danish women. Results indicated a Sn of 0.69 (95% CI 0.59–0.79) and a Sp of 0.66 (95% CI 0.64–0.68) to identify women with a BMD T score of ≤ 2.0 at the femoral neck or lumbar spine.[8]
- Retrospective validation of postmenopausal Japanese women. Results indicated a Sn of 0.90 and a Sp of 0.42 to identify women with a spinal BMD T score of ≤ –2.5 with a cutoff score of ≥ 12.[9]
- Retrospective validation of postmenopausal women from the United States. Results indicated the cutoff score should be > 7 to achieve a Sn of 0.89 (95% CI 0.84–0.94) and a Sp of 0.58 (95% CI 0.55–0.61) to identify women with BMD T scores ≤ –2.5 measured at the femoral neck.[10]

## References

1. Lydick E, Cook K, Turpin J, Melton M, Stine R, Byrnes C. Development and validation of a simple questionnaire to facilitate identification of women likely to have low bone density. *Am J Man Care*. 1998;4:37–48.
2. Cadarette SM, Jaglal SB, Murray TM. Validation of the simple calculated osteoporosis risk estimation (SCORE) for patient selection for bone densitometry. *Osteoporos Int*. 1999;10:85–90.
3. Cadarette SM, Jaglal SB, Murray TM, McIsaac WJ, Joseph L, Brown JP. Evaluation of decision rules for referring women for bone densitometry by duel-energy X-ray absorptiometry. *JAMA*. 2001;286:57–63.
4. Ben Sedrine W, Devogelaer JR, Kaufman JM, et al. Evaluation of the simple calculated osteoporosis risk estimation in a sample of Caucasian women from Belgium. *Bone*. 2001;29:374–380.

5.  Richy F, Gourlay M, Ross PD, et al. Validation and comparative evaluation of the osteoporosis self-assessment tool in a Caucasian population from Belgium. *QJM*. 2004;97:39–46.

6.  Mauck KF, Cuddihy MT, Atkinson EJ, Melton LJ III. Use of clinical prediction rules in detecting osteoporosis in a population-based sample of postmenopausal women. *Arch Intern Med*. 2005;165:530–536.

7.  Gourlay ML, Miller WC, Richy F, Garrett JM, Hanson LC, Reginster JY. Performance of osteoporosis risk assessment tools in postmenopausal women aged 45–64 years. *Osteoporos Int*. 2005;16:921–927.

8.  Rud B, Jensen JEB, Mosekilde L, Nielsen SP, Hilden J, Abrahamsen B. Performance of four clinical screening tools to select peri- and early postmenopausal women for dual X-ray absorptiometry. *Osteoporos Int*. 2005;16:764–772.

9.  Fujiwara S, Masunari N, Suzuki G, Ross PD. Performance of osteoporosis risk indices in a Japanese population. *Ther Res Clin Exp*. 2001;62:586–594.

10. Geusens P, Hochberg MC, van der Voort DJ, et al. Performance of risk indices for identifying low bone mineral density in postmenopausal women. *Mayo Clinic Proceedings*. 2002;77:629–637.

OSTEOPOROSIS

# Bone Densitometry in Women

## Osteoporosis Self-Assessment Tool (OST)[1]

**Diagnostic**

**Level: II**

Bone Densitometry
**Not** Indicated if:

Score Is ≤ **–1**

**Sensitivity 0.9**

### Predictor Variables

Equation:
$$0.2 \times (\text{weight in kg} - \text{age in years})$$

### Example of Scoring

Equation:
$$0.2 \times (\text{weight in kg} - \text{age in years}), \text{truncated to yield an integer}$$

Example: A 80-year-old woman weighs 50 kg: $0.2 \times (50 - 80) = -6$
Example: A 50-year-old woman weight 50 kg: $0.2 \times (50 - 50) = 0$

### Clinical Bottom Line

This simple sensitive equation can be used to identify patients for whom bone densitometry testing is not indicated as low bone mineral density (BMD) is unlikely. Due to the low specificity and high number of false positives, the tool cannot reliably identify patients for whom testing is indicated. This rule has been validated and may be applied to practice within the confines of the studies parameters.

### Study Specifics

*Inclusion Criteria*

- ≥ 6 months postmenopausal
- Any race or ethnic group except Caucasian
- Hip anatomy suitable for DXA scanning of the hip
- Ability to read and provide informed consent

*Exclusion Criteria*

- History or evidence of metabolic bone disease (other than postmenopausal bone loss, including but not limited to hyper- or hypoparathyroidism, Paget's disease, osteomalacia, renal osteodystrophy, osteogenesis imperfecta)
- Presence of cancer(s) with known metastasis to bone
- Evidence of significant renal impairment

- ≥ 1 ovary removed
- Bilateral hips previously fractured or replaced
- Prior use of biphosphonate, fluoride, or calcitonin

*Patient Characteristics*

- N = 860 subjects
  - 59% were Chinese, 18% were Korean, 11% were Thai, 9% were Filipino, and 4% were other
- Mean age = 62.3 (+/– 6.2)
- Prevalence of osteoporosis for Chinese women = 19%, and 7% for non-Chinese women

*Definition of Positive (Reference Standard)*

- Low BMD, diagnosed by bone densitometry, was defined as a T score at the femoral neck of ≥ 2.5 standard deviations below the mean BMD in young, healthy Asian women.

*Validation*

- Retrospective, internal validation of postmenopausal Japanese women. Results indicated a Sn of 0.98 and a Sp of 0.29 to detect a BMD T score of ≤ –2.5.[1]
- Retrospective validation of postmenopausal Japanese women. Results indicated a Sn of 0.87 and a Sp of 0.43 to identify women with a spinal BMD T score of ≤ –2.5.[2]
- Retrospective validation of perimenopausal and early postmenopausal Danish women. The cutoff score was < 2 points with a resultant Sn of 0.92 (95% CI 0.64–1.0) and a Sp of 0.71 (95% CI 0.69–0.73) to identify women with a BMD T score of ≤ 2.5 at the femoral neck.[3]
- Retrospective validation of postmenopausal women from the United States. Results indicated the cutoff score should be < 2 to achieve a Sn of 0.88 (95% CI 0.83–0.93) and a Sp of 0.52 (95% CI 0.49–0.55) to identify women with BMD T scores ≤ –2.5 measured at the femoral neck.[4]
- Retrospective validation of postmenopausal Belgian women. Results indicated an overall Sn of 0.97 and a Sp of 0.33 to identify women with a BMD T score of ≤ –2.5 at three sites (total hip, femoral neck, and L2–L4 spine).[5]
- Retrospective validation of postmenopausal Spanish women. Results indicated a Sn of 0.69 (95% CI 0.60–0.77) and a Sp of 0.59 (95% CI 0.55–0.63) to identify women with a BMD T score of ≤ –2.5 at the lumbar spine or femoral neck.[6]

## References

1. Koh LKH, Ben Sedrine W, Torralba TP, et al. A simple tool to identify Asian women at increased risk of osteoporosis. *Osteoporos Int.* 2001;12:699–705.

2. Fujiwara S, Masunari N, Suzuki G, Ross PD. Performance of osteoporosis risk indices in a Japanese population. *Ther Res Clin Exp.* 2001;62:586–594.

3. Rud B, Jensen JEB, Mosekilde L, Nielsen SP, Hilden J, Abrahemsen B. Performance of four clinical screening tools to select peri- and early postmenopausal women for dual X-ray absorptiometry. *Osteoporos Int.* 2005;16:764–772.

4. Geusens P, Hochberg MC, van der Voort DJ, et al. Performance of risk indices for identifying low bone mineral density in postmenopausal women. *Mayo Clinic Proceedings.* 2002;77:629–637.

5. Richy F, Gourlay M, Ross PD, et al. Validation and comparative evaluation of the osteoporosis self-assessment tool in a Caucasian population from Belgium. *QJM.* 2004;97:39–46.

6. Martinez-Aguila D, Gomez-Vaquero C, Rozadilla A, Romera M, Narvaez J, Nolla JM. Decision rules for selecting women for bone mineral density testing: application in postmenopausal women referred to a bone densitometry unit. *J Rheumatol.* 2007;34:1307–1312.

## OSTEOPOROSIS

# Bone Densitometry in Men

## Male Osteoporosis Risk Estimation Score (MORES)[1]

### Predictor Variables

| Risk Factor | Points |
|---|---|
| **1.** Age | |
| ≤ 55 years | 0 |
| 56–74 years | 3 |
| ≥ 75 years | 4 |
| **2.** Weight | |
| ≤ 70 kg (154 lbs) | 6 |
| 70–80 kg (155–176 lbs) | 4 |
| > 80 kg (176 lbs) | 0 |
| **3.** Chronic Obstructive Pulmonary Disease (COPD) | 3 |

**Diagnostic**

**Level: III**

Bone Densitometry **Not** Indicated if:

**Sensitivity 0.9**
(95% CI 0.8–1.0)

### Clinical Bottom Line

This CPR is a sensitive cluster of items, and individuals with ≤ 5 points can be confidently excluded from requiring bone densitometry testing as osteoporosis is unlikely. Due to the low specificity and high numbers of false positives, the tool cannot reliably identify individuals for whom testing is indicated. This rule has been validated and may be applied to practice within the confines of the study parameters; however, further external, broad studies still need to be performed.

### Study Specifics

*Inclusion Criteria*

- Noninstitutionalized, civilian males
- Ages ≥ 50

*Exclusion Criteria*

- None provided

*Patient Characteristics*

- N = 1497 subjects
  - 89% non-Hispanic white

- 8% non-Hispanic black
- 3% Hispanic
- Mean age = 63.8 (+/– 9.4)
- Prevalence of osteoporosis in derivation cohort = 5.2%

*Definition of Positive (Reference Standard)*

- Osteoporosis, diagnosed by DXA, was defined as a total hip BMD of 0.682 g/cm² or less for non-Hispanic whites, 0.723 g/cm² or less for Hispanics, and 0.751 g/cm² or less for non-Hispanic blacks. The preceding scores correspond to a T score of less than –2.5.

*Validation*

- Retrospective, internal validation of 1498 subjects from the National Health and Examination Survey III. Results indicated a Sn of 0.95 (95% CI 0.81–0.99) and a Sp of 0.61 (95% CI 0.57–0.64) to detect a bone mineral density T score of < –2.5.[1]

## References

1. Shepherd AJ, Cass AR, Carlson CA, Ray L. Development and internal validation of the male osteoporosis risk estimation score. *Ann Fam Med*. 2007;6:540–546.

## VENOUS THROMBOEMBOLISM

# Clinical Identification of Lower Extremity Deep-Vein Thrombosis (DVT)

## Wells Criteria[1]

| Probability of DVT Based on Scoring System | | |
|---|---|---|
| ≤ 0 points | Low risk | 6% probability of DVT |
| 1 or 2 points | Moderate risk | 28% probability of DVT |
| ≥ 3 | High risk | 73% probability of DVT |

**Diagnostic**

**Level: I**

### Predictor Variables

| | Score |
|---|---|
| **1.** Active cancer (treatment ongoing, within previous 6 months, or palliative) | 1 |
| **2.** Paralysis, paresis, or recent plaster immobilization of the lower extremities | 1 |
| **3.** Recently bedridden for > 3 days and/or major surgery within 4 weeks | 1 |
| **4.** Localized tenderness along the distribution of the deep venous system | 1 |
| **5.** Thigh and calf swollen | 1 |
| **6.** Calf swelling 3 cm > asymptomatic side (measured 10 cm below tibial tuberosity) | 1 |
| **7.** Pitting edema; symptomatic leg only | 1 |
| **8.** Dilated superficial veins (non-varicose) in symptomatic leg only | 1 |
| **9.** Alternative diagnosis as or more likely than DVT | −2 |

### Clinical Bottom Line

Clinical categorization of patients with suspected lower extremity (LE) deep-vein thrombosis (DVT) into high, moderate, and low probability helps determine whether a patient should be referred to a physician for further testing for the presence of a LE DVT. This rule has been extensively validated and may be applied to clinical practice within the confines of the study's parameters.

## Study Specifics

*Inclusion Criteria*

- Clinically suspected acute DVT (symptoms or signs compatible with DVT for < 60 days)

*Exclusion Criteria*

- Previous DVT or pulmonary embolism
- Contraindications to contrast media (allergy or renal insufficiency)
- Concomitant pulmonary embolism clinically suspected
- Pregnancy
- Treatment with anticoagulant therapy for more than 48 hours
- Below–knee amputation
- Patients with an alternate obvious cause for their symptoms and who had clinical features that were not compatible with DVT

*Patient Characteristics*

- N = 529 subjects
- Prevalence of LE DVT = 26%
  - 83% proximal DVT
  - 17% distal DVT

*Definition of Positive (Reference Standard)*

- Proximal or distal DVT was diagnosed by impedance plethysmography and venography

*Validation/Impact Analysis*

- Prospective validation of Canadian patients with suspected LE DVT presenting to the ED. Patient categorization and subsequent ultrasound/venography testing revealed 3.2% (95% CI 1.2–6.7) of individuals in the low category, 14.3% (95% CI 8.3–22.4) in the moderate category, and 49.0% (95% CI 34.6–63.6) in the high category were confirmed to have a DVT, thus agreeing with the ability of the low categorization to rule out DVT.[2]
- Retrospective validation in a Swiss population. The accuracy of the risk stratification/clinical probability assessment was found to be excellent as the prevalence of DVT was reported as 3.2% (95% CI 0.9–7.9), 19.4% (95% CI 12.1–28.6), and 73.9% (95% CI 58.9–85.7) in the low, moderate, and high categories, respectively.[3]

- Prospective validation of ED patients with a suspected LE DVT. All patients with DVTs were stratified according to risk. The sensitivity of pretest probability (risk stratification) and D-dimer testing was 100%, which fell to 80% when D-dimer testing was performed without stratification. The screening algorithm utilized in this study (high risk = direct venous duplex imaging (VDI), D-dimer for low and moderate risk with a follow-up VDI for positive results) has been shown to eliminate 23% of VDI tests and reduce charges by 16% while maintaining high diagnostic accuracy.[4]
- Prospective validation of patients with suspected LE DVT. In the high-probability group, 71% of individuals had a DVT, 28% of patients in the moderate–probability group had a DVT, and 0% of individuals in the low-risk group had a DVT.[5]
- Prospective validation of Swiss patients with suspected LE DVT. In the low-risk category, 13.0% (95% CI 7.0–9.0) of patients were diagnosed with a DVT, 30.0% (95% CI 22.0–38.0) were in the moderate-risk category, and 67.0% (95% CI 54.0–70.0) were in the high-risk category, indicating the need for additional testing beyond stratification. By combining D-dimer testing with low-risk stratification, a negative predictive value of 100% was found; thus, 10% of ultrasound tests could have been eliminated with individuals in this category.[6]
- Prospective validation of patients presenting to the ED with suspected proximal LE DVT. Of individuals categorized as low probability, 8.0% (95% CI 7.0-10.0) were diagnosed with a DVT, 27.0% (95% CI 23.0–31.0) of individuals categorized as moderate probability were diagnosed with a DVT, and 66% (95% CI 61.0–71.0) of individuals in the high-probability category were diagnosed with a DVT. If an individual categorized as low probability had a negative ultrasound, only 1.6% of DVTs were missed. A low-pretest probability and a negative D-dimer test also missed only 1.8% of DVTs.[7]
- Prospective validation of ED patients suspected of possessing a LE DVT. Of individuals categorized as low probability, 2.0% (95% CI 0.1–11.0) were diagnosed with a DVT, 14.0% (95% CI 4.0–24.0) of those with a moderate probability were diagnosed with a DVT, and 59.0% (95% CI 35.0–82.0) of individuals with a high probability were diagnosed with a DVT.[8]
- Prospective validation of Canadian patients presenting to the ED with suspected proximal LE DVT. A musculoskeletal condition as a primary diagnosis was found in 9.3% of patients. Of individuals categorized as low probability, 4.5% (95% CI 2.7–6.8) were diagnosed with a DVT, 18.8% (95% CI 15.2–22.8) of those with a moderate probability were diagnosed

with a DVT, and 47.3% (95% CI 40.2–54.4) of individuals with a high probability were diagnosed with a DVT. Low-risk stratification and a negative D-dimer test resulted in 1% of patients diagnosed with a DVT.[9]

- Prospective validation of an outpatient cohort with suspected LE DVT. Of patients categorized as low probability, 6% were diagnosed with a DVT, 20% of patients categorized as moderate probability were diagnosed with a DVT, and 69% of patients categorized with high probability were diagnosed with a DVT.[10]

- Retrospective validation of outpatients with a suspected proximal DVT and various musculoskeletal disorders. Of individuals categorized as low probability, 6% were diagnosed with a DVT, 14% of those with a moderate probability were diagnosed with a DVT, and 47% of individuals with a high probability were diagnosed with a DVT. The probability of patients with fractures, surgery, or traumatic injuries developing venous thromboembolisms were as follows: low probability was 11%, moderate probability was 15%, and high probability was 50%.[11]

## References

1. Wells PS, Hirsh J, Anderson DR, et al. A simple clinical model for the diagnosis of deep-vein thrombosis combined with impedance plethysmography: potential for an improvement in the diagnostic process. *J Intern Med*. 1998;243:15–23.

2. Anderson DR, Wells PS, Philip S, et al. Thrombosis in the emergency department: use of a clinical diagnosis model to safely avoid the need for urgent radiological investigation. *Arch Intern Med*. 1999;159:477–482.

3. Miron MJ, Perrier A, Bounameaux H. Clinical assessment of suspected deep vein thrombosis: comparison between a score and clinical assessment. *J Intern Med*. 2000;247:249–254.

4. Dryjski M, O'Brien-Irr MS, Harris LM, Hassett J, Janicke D. Evaluation of a screening protocol to exclude the diagnosis of deep venous thrombosis among emergency department patients. *J Vasc Surg*. 2001;34:1010–1015.

5. Funfsinn N, Calieze C, Demarmels Biasiutti F, et al. Rapid D-dimer testing and pre-test probability in the exclusion of deep venous thrombosis in symptomatic outpatients. *Blood Coagul Fibrinolysis*. 2001;12:165–170.

6. Cornuz J, Ghali WA, Hayoz D, Stoianov R, Depairon M, Yersin B. Clinical prediction of deep vein thrombosis using two risk assessment methods in combination with rapid quantitative D-dimer testing. *Am J Med*. 2002;112:198–203.

7. Kraaijenhagen RA, Piovella F, Bernardi E, et al. Simplification of the diagnostic management of deep vein thrombosis. *Arch Intern Med*. 2002;162:907–911.

8. Shields GP, Turnipseed S, Panacek EA, Melnikoff N, Gosselin R, White RH. Validation of the Canadian clinical probability model for acute venous thrombosis. *Acad Emerg Med*. 2002;9:561–566.

9. Anderson DR, Kovacs MJ, Stiell I, et al. Combined use of clinical assessment and D-dimer to improve the management of patients presenting to the emergency department with suspected deep vein thrombosis (the *edited* study). *J Thromb Haemost*. 2003;1:645–651.

10. Constans J, Boutinet C, Salmi R, et al. Comparison of four clinical prediction scores for the diagnosis of lower limb deep vein thrombosis in outpatients. *Am J Med.* 2003:115:436–440.
11. Riddle DL, Hopener MR, Kraaijenhagen RA, Anderson J, Wells PS. Preliminary validation of clinical assessment for deep vein thrombosis in orthopaedic outpatients. *Clin Orthop Related Res.* 2005;432:252–257.

VENOUS THROMBOEMBOLISM

# Percent Probability of an Upper Extremity Deep-Vein Thrombosis (DVT)[1]

| Diagnostic | Probability of UE DVT | | |
|---|---|---|---|
| | ≤ 0 points | Low probability | 12% (95% CI 10–23) probability |
| **Level: II** | 1 point | Intermediate probability | 20% (95% CI 9–30) probability |
| | 2+ points | High probability | 70% (95% CI 57–83) probability |

## Predictor Variables

| | Score |
|---|---|
| **1.** The presence of venous material (catheter or access device in a subclavian or jugular vein, or a pacemaker) | 1 |
| **2.** Pitting edema | 1 |
| **3.** Localized pain in the upper limb | 1 |
| **4.** Another diagnosis is at least as plausible as DVT | −1 |

## Clinical Bottom Line

Clinical categorization of patients with suspected upper extremity (UE) DVT into high, intermediate, and low probability will help to determine whether a patient should be referred to a physician for further testing for the presence of UE DVT. The CPR has undergone both internal as well as external validation; however, they were incorporated into the same study. It may be applied to clinical practice within the confines of the study's parameters.

## Study Specifics

### Inclusion Criteria

- Patients hospitalized who were referred to the vascular exploration unit for suspicion of UE DVT

### Exclusion Criteria

- None reported

*Patient Characteristics*

- N = 140 subjects
- Prevalence of UE DVT = 36%
- Mean age = 59 (+/− 18)
- Gender
  - Female = 48%
  - Male = 52%

*Definition of Positive (Reference Standard)*

- UE DVT was diagnosed by B-mode compression ultrasound and color Doppler investigation of the radial, brachial, ulnar, axillary, subclavian, and internal jugular veins

*Validation/Impact Analysis*

- Prospective internal validation of the scoring system. Results found that 9% of patients with a score of 0 or less had UE DVT, 37% with a score of 1 had UE DVT, and 64% with a score of 2 or greater had UE DVT.[1]
- Prospective external validation. Results found that 13% of patients with a score of 0 or less had UE DVT, 38% with a score of 1 had UE DVT, and 69% with a score of 2 or greater had UE DVT.[1]

## References

1. Constans J, Salmi LR, Sevestre-Pietri MA, et al. A clinical prediction score for upper extremity deep venous thrombosis. *Thromb Haemost.* 2008;99:202–207.

VENOUS THROMBOEMBOLISM

# Clinical Identification of Pulmonary Embolism (PE)

## Wells Score[1]

| Diagnostic | **Probability of PE** | | |
|---|---|---|---|
| **Level: II** | < 2.0 points | Low risk | 3.6% probability of PE |
| | 2.0 to 6.0 points | Moderate risk | 20.5% probability of PE |
| | > 6.0 points | High risk | 66.7% probability of PE |

## Predictor Variables

|  | | Score |
|---|---|---|
| **1.** | Clinical signs and symptoms of DVT (minimum of leg swelling and pain with palpation of the deep veins) | 3.0 |
| **2.** | No alternative diagnosis | 3.0 |
| **3.** | Heart rate > 100 bpm | 1.5 |
| **4.** | Immobilization of surgery in the previous 4 weeks | 1.5 |
| **5.** | Previous DVT/PE | 1.5 |
| **6.** | Hemoptysis | 1.0 |
| **7.** | Malignancy (on treatment, treated in the last 6 months, or palliative) | 1.0 |

## Clinical Bottom Line

Clinical categorization of patients with suspected pulmonary embolism (PE) into low, moderate, and high probability will help to determine whether a patient should be referred to a physician for further testing for the presence of a PE. This rule has been extensively validated and may be applied to clinical practice within the confines of the study's parameters.

## Study Specifics

*Inclusion Criteria[2]*

- Suspected pulmonary embolism
- Symptoms < 30 days

*Exclusion Criteria[2]*

- Suspected UE DVT as source of PE
- No symptoms of PE for > 3 days
- Use of anticoagulation for > 72 hours
- Expected survival of < 3 months
- Contraindications to contrast media
- Pregnancy
- Geographic inaccessibility precluding follow-up
- < 18 years old
- Inability to obtain permission from the patient or patient's attending physician

*Patient Characteristics*

- N = 1260 subjects
- Prevalence of PE = 17.6%

*Definition of Positive (Reference Standard)*

- PE was diagnosed by venography, pulmonary angiography, ultrasound, and Ventilation/Perfusion scan (VQ scans).

*Validation/Impact Analysis*

- Retrospective validation of Canadian inpatients and outpatients present-ing with symptoms of PE. Of patients placed in the low-pretest probability category, 2% (95% CI 0.2–7.1) were diagnosed with a PE, 18.8% (95% CI 12.4–26.6) of patients placed in the moderate-pretest probability category were diagnosed with a PE, and 50% (95% CI 27.2–72.8) of patients placed in the high-pretest probability category were diagnosed with a PE. The dichotomized rule was defined as "PE Unlikely": a score of ≤ 4.0, and "PE Likely": a score of > 4.0. Of patients categorized as "PE Unlikely," 5.1% (95% CI 2.3–9.4) were diagnosed with a PE, and 39.1% (95% CI 27.6–51.6) were diagnosed in the "PE Likely" group. A low-pretest probability score combined with a negative D-dimer test produced a 1.7% missed PE rate.[1]
- Prospective validation of Swiss or French patients presenting to their respec-tive EDs with a suspicion of PE. Of patients placed in the low-pretest prob-ability category, 12% (95% CI 7–17) were diagnosed with a PE, 40% (95% CI 31–50) of patients placed in the moderate-pretest probability category were diagnosed with a PE, and 91% (95% CI 59–100) of patients placed in the high-pretest probability category were diagnosed with a PE.[3]

- Retrospective validation of inpatients and outpatients from a large military-based health care system. Of patients placed in the low-pretest probability category, 15.3% (95% CI 9.5–23.7) were diagnosed with a PE, 34.8% (95% CI 27.9–42.4) of patients placed in the moderate-pretest probability category were diagnosed with a PE, and 47.2% (95% CI 32.0–63.0) of patients placed in the high-pretest probability category were diagnosed with a PE. Odds ratios for PE were calculated at 2.95 (95% CI 1.56–5.59) in the moderate-pretest probability group and 4.95 (95% CI 2.11–11.64) in the high-probability group as compared to the low-probability group.[4]

- Prospective validation of predominately managed-care patients, presenting to the ED with suspected PE. Physicians, residents, and physician assistants all collected data. Additional exclusion criteria included > 85 years old and > 350 lbs. Of patients placed in the low-pretest probability category, 2% (95% CI 0–9) were diagnosed with a PE, 15% (95% CI 7–26) of patients placed in the moderate-pretest probability category were diagnosed with a PE, and 43% (95% CI 18–71) of patients placed in the high-pretest probability category were diagnosed with a PE. Patients were also dichotomized into PE Likely and PE Unlikely categories with 3% (95% CI 0–9) of patients in the PE Unlikely probability diagnosed with PE and 28% (95% CI 18–71) of patients in the PE Likely probability group diagnosed with PE.[5]

- Prospective validation of Dutch inpatients (18%) and outpatients (82%) presenting to the ED with suspected PE. Of patients categorized as PE Unlikely with a negative D-dimer test, 0.5% (95% CI 0.2–1.1) were later diagnosed with a PE by a CT scan.[6]

- Prospective validation of Belgian patients presenting to the ED with a suspicion of PE. Of patients placed in the low-pretest probability category by physicians in training, 3% (95% CI 1–9) were diagnosed with a PE, as compared to 2% (95% CI 1–7) diagnosed by the supervising physicians; 31% (95% CI 22–42) of patients placed in the moderate-pretest probability category by physicians in training were diagnosed with a PE, as compared to 33% (95% CI 23–44) by the supervision phsyicians. Of patients placed in the high-pretest probability category by supervising physicians, 100% (95% CI 61–100) were diagnosed with a PE, as compared to 100% (95% CI 65–100) by the physicians in training. The Wells "Dichotomized" Rule was also analyzed with regard to diagnosed PEs between physicians in training and the supervising physicians. Of patients placed in the PE Unlikely category (≤ 4 points), 9% (95% CI 5–15) were diagnosed with PE by the physicians in training vs 7% (95% CI 4–12) by the supervising physicians;

49% (95% CI 35–63) of patients placed in the PE Likely category (> 4 points) were diagnosed with PE by the physicians in training vs 59% (95% CI 43–72) by the supervising physicians.[7]

- Prospective validation of Turkish patients presenting to the ED as well as inpatients suspected of having a PE. Of patients placed in the low-pretest probability category, 7.8% were diagnosed with a PE, 26.4% of patients placed in the moderate-pretest probability category were diagnosed with a PE, and 89.6% of patients placed in the high-pretest probability category were diagnosed with a PE by CT angiography and/or venography.[8]

## References

1. Wells PS, Anderson DR, Rodger M, et al. Derivation of a simple clinical model to categorize patient's probability of pulmonary embolism: increasing the model's utility with the SimpliRed D-dimer. *Thromb Haemost.* 2000;83:416–420.

2. Wells PS, Ginsberg JS, Anderson DR, et al. Use of a clinical model for safe management of patients with suspected pulmonary embolism. *Ann Intern Med.* 1998;129:997–1005.

3. Chagnon I, Bounameaux H, Aujesky D, et al. Comparison of two clinical prediction rules and implicit assessment among patients with suspected pulmonary embolism. *Am J Med.* 2002;113:269–275.

4. Moores LK, Collen JF, Woods KM, Shorr AF. Practical utility of clinical prediction rules for suspected pulmonary embolism in a large academic institution. *Thromb Res.* 2004;113:1–6.

5. Wolf SJ, McCubbin TR, Feldhaus KM, Faragher JP, Adcock DM. Prospective validation of Wells criteria in the evaluation of patients with suspected pulmonary embolism. *Ann Emerg Med.* 2004;44:503–510.

6. van Belle A, Buller HR, Hisman HV, et al. Effectiveness of managing suspected pulmonary embolism using an algorithm combining clinical probability D-dimer testing, and computed tomography. *JAMA.* 2006;295:172–179.

7. Penaloza A, Melot C, Dochy E, et al. Assessment of pretest probability of pulmonary embolism in the emergency department by physicians in training using the Wells model. *Thrombosis Research.* 2007;120:173–179.

8. Calisir C, Yavas US, Ozkan IR, et al. Performance of the Wells and revised Geneva scores for predicting pulmonary embolism. *Eur J Emerg Med.* 2009;16:49–52.

VENOUS THROMBOEMBOLISM

# Determining Probability for Pulmonary Embolism (PE)

## The Revised Geneva Score[1]

| Diagnostic | Clinical Pretest Probability of PE | | |
|---|---|---|---|
| | 0–3 points | Low probability | 9% probability of PE |
| Level: II | 4–10 points | Intermediate probability | 28% probability of PE |
| | ≥ 11 points | High probability | 72% probability of PE |

### Predictor Variables

| | Score |
|---|---|
| **1.** Age > 65 years old | 1 |
| **2.** Previous DVT or pulmonary embolism (PE) | 3 |
| **3.** Surgery (under general anesthesia) or fracture (lower limbs) within 1 month | 2 |
| **4.** Active or malignant condition (solid or hematologic malignant condition, currently active or considered cured < 1 year) | 2 |
| **5.** Unilateral lower limb pain | 3 |
| **6.** Hemoptysis | 2 |
| **7.** Heart rate: 75–94 beats per minute | 3 |
|                 ≥ 95 beats per minute | 5 |
| **8.** Pain on lower limb deep venous palpation and unilateral edema | 4 |

### Clinical Bottom Line

Clinical categorization of patients with suspected PE into high, intermediate, and low probability will help to determine whether a patient should be referred to a physician for further testing for the presence of a PE. This rule has been extensively validated and may be applied to clinical practice within the confines of the study's parameters.

## Study Specifics

*Inclusion Criteria*

- Suspected PE
  - Defined as acute onset of new or worsening shortness of breath or chest pain without no other obvious cause

*Exclusion Criteria*

- Ongoing anticoagulant therapy
- Contraindications to CT scans
  - Known allergies to contrast, <0.5 mL/s creatinine clearance, or pregnancy
- Suspected massive PE with shock
- < 3 months of expected life expectancy

*Patient Characteristics*

- N = 965 subjects
- Mean age = 60.6 (+/− 19.4)
- Prevalence of pulmonary embolism = 23%
- Gender
  - Female = 58%
  - Male = 42%

*Definition of Positive (Reference Standard)*

- PE was diagnosed by a proximal DVT on ultrasonography, or a positive helical CT scan, pulmonary angiogram, or ventilation-perfusion lung scan.

*Validation*

- Retrospective, internal and external validation of Swiss patients presenting to the ED with suspected pulmonary embolism. Of patients with PE, 7.9% (95% CI 5.0–12.1) were categorized as low probability, 28.5% (95% CI 24.6–32.8) of patients with PE were categorized as intermediate probability, and 73.7% (95% CI 61.0–83.4) were categorized as high probability.[1]
- Retrospective validation and comparison to the Wells Rule in patients with a suspected pulmonary embolism. The Revised Geneva Score performed equally as well as the Wells Rule with a finding of 8.3% (95% CI 4.0–12.7) of patients in the low-probability category diagnosed with a PE, 22.8% (95% CI 14.7–29.9) of patients in the intermediate-probability category

diagnosed with a PE, and 71.4% (95% CI 35.3-100) of patients in the high-probability category diagnosed with a PE. At the 3-month mark, no individuals categorized as low or intermediate probability and with a negative D-dimer test were diagnosed with a venous thromboembolism.[2]

- Prospective validation of Turkish patients presenting to the ED as well as inpatients suspected of having a PE. Of patients placed in the low-pretest probability category, 0% were diagnosed with a PE, 25.6% of patients placed in the intermediate-pretest probability category were diagnosed with a PE, and 83.3% of patients placed in the high-pretest probability category were diagnosed with a PE by CT angiography and/or venography.[3]

*Impact Analysis*

- None to date

## References

1. Le Gal G, Righini M, Roy PM, et al. Prediction of pulmonary embolism in the emergency department: the revised Geneva score. *Ann Intern Med.* 2006;144:165–171.
2. Klok FA, Kruisman E, Spaan J, et al. Comparison of the revised Geneva score with the Wells rule for assessing clinical probability of pulmonary embolism. *J Thromb Haemost.* 2008;6:40–44.
3. Calisir C, Yavas US, Ozkan IR, et al. Performance of the Wells and revised Geneva scores for predicting pulmonary embolism. *Eur J Emerg Med.* 2009;16:49–52.

PERIPHERAL NEUROPATHY

# Clinical Identification of Peripheral Neuropathy Among Older Persons[1]

## Predictor Variables

**1.** Absence of an Achilles' reflex
**2.** Decreased vibration sensation
**3.** Decreased position sense at the toe

## Clinical Bottom Line

Subjects that possess two or more predictor variables have a moderate shift in probability for the presence of peripheral neuropathy as compared to electrodiagnostic testing. A methodological quality analysis is suggested before implementing this CPR as a component of the best available evidence.

## Examination

- Absence of an Achilles' reflex (**Figure 4.8**)
  - Tested via tendon striking and plantar surface striking with and without facilitation (slight plantar flexion, eyes closed tight, and pulling clasped hands apart).

| **Diagnostic** |
| --- |
| **Level: IV** |
| Diagnostic for Peripheral Neuropathy if: |
| **Two or More** Predictor Variables Present |
| **+LR 5.9** |

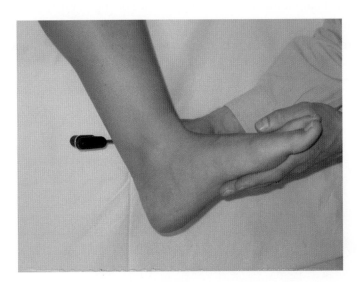

**Figure 4.8**
Achilles' reflex.

- Decreased vibration sensation (**Figure 4.9**)
  - A 128-Hz tuning fork was maximally struck and placed just proximal to the nail bed of the first digit of the great toe. The patient indicated "gone" when the vibration was no longer sensed and the time was recorded in seconds. Decreased vibration sensation was defined as < 8 seconds.

**Figure 4.9**
Assessment of vibration sensation.

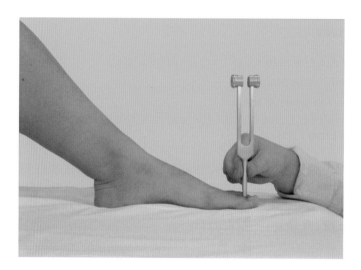

- Decreased position sense at the toe (**Figure 4.10**)
  - The great toe is held at the medial and lateral surfaces by the examiner's thumb and forefinger. A series of 10 randomly administered movements were administered with the subject's eyes closed. Each movement was a smooth small amplitude motion over a distance of approximately 1 cm and over a time frame of 1 second. Decreased position sense was defined as correctly perceiving the direction of motion fewer than 8 out of 10 times.

**Figure 4.10**
Assessment of position sense of the great toe.

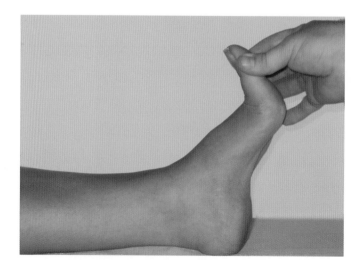

## Study Specifics

*Inclusion Criteria*

- Ages 50–80
- Electrodiagnostic evidence of a diffuse, primarily axonal peripheral polyneu-ropathy (neuropathy group)
  - Normal electrodiagnostic studies (control group)

*Patient Characteristics*

- N = 100 subjects
- Mean age of patients with neuropathy = 65.6 (+/– 9.0)
- Prevalence of peripheral neuropathy = 68%
- Gender
  - Female = 37%
  - Male = 63%

*Definition of Positive (Reference Standard)*

- Electrodiagnostic evidence of diffuse, primarily axonal peripheral polyneuropathy

*Validation/Impact Analysis*

- None reported to date

## References

1. Richardson JK. The clinical identification of peripheral neuropathy among older persons. *Arch Phys Med Rehabil.* 2002;83:1553–1558.

# CHAPTER 5

# CERVICOTHORACIC REGION AND TEMPOROMANDIBULAR JOINT

## DIAGNOSTIC

# Diagnosis of Cervical Radiculopathy[1]

**Diagnostic**

**Level: IV**

Diagnostic for Cervical Radiculopathy if:

**Three or More** Predictor Variables Present

**+LR 6.1** (95% CI 2.0–18.6)

### Predictor Variables

1. Cervical rotation toward the involved side < 60°
2. Positive upper-limb tension test A (ULTT A)
3. Positive cervical distraction test
4. Positive Spurling's A test

### Clinical Bottom Line

The presence of three or more predictor variables indicates a moderate shift in probability that a patient will test positive for cervical radiculopathy using needle electromyography. A methodological quality analysis is suggested before implementing this CPR as a component of the best available evidence.

### Examination

- Cervical rotation toward the involved side less than 60° (**Figure 5.1**)
  - The patient was placed in sitting position. The clinician stood over the patient and the goniometer was aligned over the shoulder and the nose. The patient was asked to rotate toward the involved side as far as possible and the measurement was taken.

**Figure 5.1**
Cervical rotation ROM.

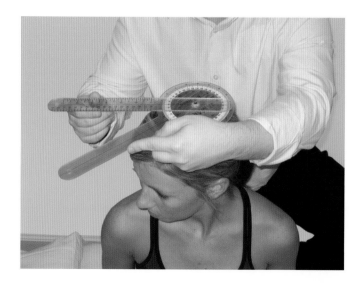

- ULTT A (**Figure 5.2**)
  - Step 1           Scapular depression
  - Step 2           Shoulder abduction
  - Step 3           Forearm supination, wrist and finger extension
  - Step 4           Shoulder lateral rotation
  - Step 5           Elbow extension
  - Step 6A         Contralateral cervical side bending
  - Step 6B         Ipsilateral cervical side bending
- Positive if patient's symptoms are reproduced, a side-to-side difference of > 10° in elbow extension, or symptoms increased in Step 6A or decreased in Step 6B.

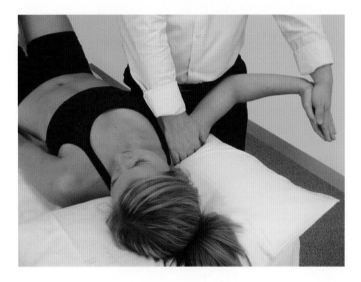

**Figure 5.2**
Upper-limb tension test A.

**Figure 5.3**
(Below) Cervical distraction test.

- Cervical distraction test (**Figure 5.3**)
  - The patient was positioned in the supine position. The clinician grasped the chin and occiput, flexed the patient's neck to position of comfort, and gradually applied a distraction force up to ~14 kg. The test was considered positive if patient's symptoms decreased.

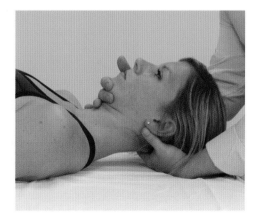

- Spurling's A test (**Figure 5.4**)
  - ▪ The patient was positioned in the sitting position. The neck was passively side bent toward the symptomatic side and ~7 kg of overpressure was applied. The test was considered positive if the patient's symptoms were reproduced.

**Figure 5.4**
Spurling's A test.

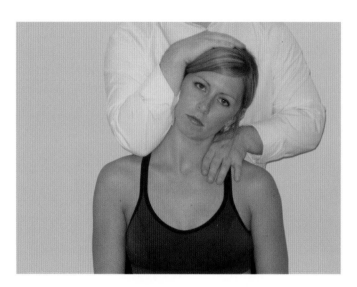

## Study Specifics

### Inclusion Criteria

- Ages 18–70
- Referred to the electrophysiologic laboratories with suspected cervical radiculopathy or carpal tunnel syndrome (CTS) as judged by the electrophysiologic laboratory provider

### Exclusion Criteria

- Systemic disease known to cause generalized peripheral neuropathy
- Primary report of bilateral radiating arm pain
- History of upper-extremity conditions on the involved side that may affect the patient's level of function
- Discontinuation of work more than 6 months because of the condition
- History of surgical procedures for pathologies giving rise to neck pain or CTS

- Previous needle electromyography (EMG) and nerve conduction study (NCS) testing the symptomatic limb or cervical radiculopathy, CTS, or both
- Workers' compensation received or pending litigation for condition

*Patient Characteristics*

- N = 82 subjects
- Prevalence of cervical radiculopathy = 23%
- Mean age = 45 (+/− 12)
- Gender
  - Female = 50%
  - Male = 50%

*Definition of Positive (Reference Standard)*

- Diagnosis of cervical radiculopathy using needle EMG

*Validation/Impact Analysis*

- None reported to date

## References

1. Wainner RS, Fritz JM, Irrgang JJ, Boninger ML, Delitto A, Allison S. Reliability and diagnostic accuracy of the clinical examination and patient self-report measures for cervical radiculopathy. *Spine*. 2003;28:52–62.

PROGNOSTIC

# Prediction of Persistent Whiplash-Associated Disorders (WAD)[1]

**Prognostic**

**Level: IV**

**Quality Score: 61%**

Prognostic for
**Not** Having
Persistent Disability if:

Categorized as
**Low Risk** Using
the Questions at Right

**–LR 0.2**

## Predictor Variables

Question 1: "Did the collision occur at a location other than an intersection in the city?"

Question 2: "Have you experienced upper back pain since the collision?"

*Yes* to both questions indicates **high risk** for 6-month WAD.

*No* to both questions; patient is asked one additional question:

Question 3: "Do you still experience neck pain (2-weeks post injury)?"

*No* to Question 3 indicates **low risk**.

*Yes* to Question 3 indicates **high risk**.

Those who answered "Yes" to one of the first two questions and "No" to the third question are then asked:

Question 4: "Do you still experience shoulder pain (2-weeks post injury)?"

*No* to Question 4 indicates **low risk**.

*Yes* to Question 4 indicates **high risk**.

## Clinical Bottom Line

This clinical rule allows for early prediction (within 2 weeks of the motor vehicle collision) of not having long-term (6 months) dysfunction categorized as WAD stage 3+ (see Definition of Positive). Individuals who are categorized as "low risk" have a moderate shift in probability (8% chance) of not having a WAD at 6 months. The methodological quality of this study is below the suggested standard, so results should be taken with caution if this CPR is used clinically before validation.

## Study Specifics

*Inclusion Criteria (from Original Study)[2]*

- Ages ≥ 18
- Involved in a rear-end motor vehicle collision, in which the vehicle was hit from behind
- Ability to answer questions in English
- First visit to the ED for the injury in question

*Exclusion Criteria (from Original Study)[2]*

- Diagnosed with a fracture, dislocation, or subluxation of the vertebrae
- Injury to the spinal column
- Head injury

*Patient Characteristics (from Original Study)[2]*

- N = 353 subjects
- Percentage of subjects with persistent WAD = 35.3%
- Gender
  - Female = 63.5%
  - Male = 36.5%
- Driver of vehicle = 73.9%
- Car was stopped = 77.3%
- Looking straight ahead = 64.3%

*Definition of Positive (Reference Standard)*

- WAD was defined as the presence of either neck pain, upper back pain, or shoulder pain that met the level of pain and frequency indicated at stages 3+ at 6 months post motor vehicle accident (MVA).
- Definitions
  - Frequency: occasional (< once a week), regular (once a week or more), daily
  - Severity: none, minor (a nuisance), moderate (affects one's regular activities or work), severe (a significant handicap to regular work or activities)
- Grading
  - 0 = No symptoms
  - 1 = Minor pain of occasional frequency
  - 2 = Moderate pain of occasional frequency or minor pain of regular or daily frequency
  - 3 = Moderate pain of regular frequency or severe pain of occasional frequency
  - 4 = Moderate pain of daily frequency or severe pain of regular frequency
  - 5 = Severe pain of daily frequency

*Validation/Impact Analysis*

- None reported to date

## References

1. Hartling L, Pickett W, Brison RJ. Derivation of a clinical decision rule for whiplash associated disorders among individuals involved in rear-end collisions. *Accid Ana Prev*. 2002;34:531–539.
2. Brison RJ, Hartling L, Pickett W. A prospective study of acceleration-extension injuries following rear-end motor vehicle collisions. *J Musculoskeletal Pain*. 2000;8:97–113.

PROGNOSTIC

# Predicting Short-Term Outcomes with Cervical Radiculopathy[1]

**Prognostic**

**Level: IV**

**Quality Score: 72%**

A Successful Outcome Likely if:

**Three or More** Predictor Variables Present

**+LR 5.2** (95% CI 2.4–11.3)

## Predictor Variables

**1.** Age < 54
**2.** Dominant arm is not affected
**3.** Looking down does not worsen symptoms
**4.** Received multimodal treatment for ≥ 50% of visits
   **a.** Manual therapy (muscle energy, mobilization, or manipulation to the cervical or thoracic spine)
   **b.** Cervical traction (manual or mechanical)
   **c.** Deep-neck flexor muscle strengthening

## Clinical Bottom Line

There is a moderate shift in probability that patients with cervical radiculopathy who possess three or more predictor variables will have a clinically meaningful change in neck disability, specific functional activities, pain, or overall improvement at a 4-week follow-up. The methodological quality of the derivation study was acceptable; therefore, it is appropriate to use this CPR as a component of the best available evidence.

## Study Specifics

*Inclusion Criteria*

- All four criteria for cervical radiculopathy
  - Cervical rotation toward the symptomatic of < 60°
  - Spurling's A test
  - Upper-limb tension test A
  - Cervical distraction test
- Read and understand English to complete the outcome measures
- Complete self-report measures at intake and follow-up

*Exclusion Criteria*

- None reported

*Patient Characteristics*

- N = 96 subjects
- Mean age = 50.8 (+/− 9.5)
- Percentage of subjects considered a treatment success = 53%
- Gender
  - Female = 64%
  - Male = 36%
- Mean number of visits = 6.4 (+/− 1.7)
- Mean duration of treatment (days) = 28 (+/− 9)

*Definition of Success*

- Surpassing the minimally clinically important change (MCIC) for all four outcome measures
  - Neck Disability Index (MCIC = 7 points)
  - Patient Specific Functional Scale (MCIC = 2 points)
  - Numerical Pain Rating Scale (MCIC = 2 points)
  - Global Rating of Change Scale (≥ +5, moderate perceived change)

*Validation/Impact Analysis*

- None reported to date

## References

1. Cleland JA, Fritz JM, Whitman JM, Heath R. Predictors of short-term outcome in people with a clinical diagnosis of cervical radiculopathy. *Phys Ther*. 2007;87:1619–1632.

INTERVENTIONAL

# Cervical Manipulation for Mechanical Neck Pain[1]

**Interventional**

**Level: IV**

**Quality Score 61%**

Cervical Manipulation Indicated if:

**Four or More** Predictor Variables Present

**+LR 5.3** (95% CI 1.7–16.5)

## Predictor Variables

1. Initial Neck Disability Index score < 11.50 points
2. Bilateral pattern of involvement
3. Not performing sedentary work > 5 hours/day
4. Feels better while moving the neck
5. Does not feel worse while extending the neck
6. Diagnosis of spondylosis without radiculopathy

## Clinical Bottom Line

The presence of four or more predictor variables indicates a moderate shift in probability that a patient would either experience a ≥ 50% reduction in pain, report a moderate or higher level of improvement, or report being "very satisfied" immediately after cervical manipulation. The methodological quality of the derivation study was acceptable; therefore, it is appropriate to use this CPR as a component of the best available evidence.

## Intervention

Patients were treated for one session. Treatment included:

- Cervical manipulation (**Figure 5.5**)
  - The clinician stood at the head of the bed with the patient in the supine position. The clinician held the patient's head in a cradle position. A side-gliding motion assessment was introduced from the occiput to C7 to identify the hypomobile segments. The clinician then side bent the cervical spine down to the hypomobile segment, flexed down to the hypomobile segment, and rotated away until the segment began to move. The thrust was applied up and away from the segment, in a direction toward the opposite eye. The technique was applied one time per hypomobile segment.

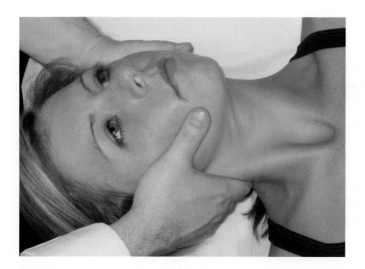

**Figure 5.5**
Supine mid-cervical upglide manipulation.

## Study Specifics

*Inclusion Criteria*

- Diagnosis
  - Cervical spondylosis with or without radiculopathy
  - Herniated disc of the cervical spine
  - Myofascial pain syndrome
  - Cervicogenic headache

*Exclusion Criteria*

- Vertebral basilar insufficiency (symptoms of nystagmus, dizziness, lightheadedness, or visual disturbances)
- Progressive neurological deficits
- Severe osteoporosis
- History of cervical fracture or surgery
- Diagnosis of psychological disorders
- Systemic diseases
- Other contraindications to cervical manipulation

*Patient Characteristics*

- N = 100 subjects
- Mean age = 46 (+/– 11)
- Percentage of subjects considered a treatment success = 60%

- Gender
  - Female = 66%
  - Male = 34%
- Chronic (> 3 months) = 43%
- Subacute (3 weeks – 3 months) = 24%
- Acute (< 3 weeks) = 32%

*Definition of Success*

- ≥ 50% pain reduction on the Numerical Pain Rating Scale (NPRS) *or*
- ≥ 4 on the Global Rating of Change Scale (GROC) *or*
- Report of "very satisfied" on the satisfaction scale

*Validation/Impact Analysis*

- None reported to date

## References

1. Tseng YL, Wang WTJ, Chen WY, Tsun-Jen H, Tzu-Ching C, Fu-Kong L. Predictors for the immediate responders to cervical manipulation in patients with neck pain. *Man Ther*. 2006;306–315.

INTERVENTIONAL

# Thoracic Manipulation for Mechanical Neck Pain[1]

**Interventional**

**Level: IV**

Thoracic Manipulation Indicated if:

**Three or More** Predictor Variables Present

**+LR 5.5** (95% CI 2.7–12.0)

## Predictor Variables

1. Symptoms < 30 days
2. No symptoms distal to the shoulder
3. Looking up does not aggravate symptoms
4. Fear Avoidance Belief Questionnaire - Physical Activity subscale < 12
5. Diminished upper-thoracic spine (T3–T5) kyphosis
6. Cervical extension range of motion (ROM) < 30°

## Clinical Bottom Line

Patients with cervical spine pain and three or more of the above findings are likely to experience moderate perceived global improvement from thoracic spine manipulation and cervical ROM exercise within two treatment sessions (4–8 days). The methodological quality of the derivation study was acceptable; therefore, it is appropriate to use this CPR as a component of the best available evidence.

## Examination

- Diminished upper-thoracic spine (T3–T5) kyphosis:
  - The variable was considered positive if the normal thoracic kyphosis was noted to be flattening of the convexity of the T3–T5 segments
- Cervical extension ROM < 30° (**Figure 5.6**)
  - The patient was in the sitting position. An inclinometer was placed on the top of the head and zeroed. The patient was asked to actively extend his or her neck and the measurement was taken.

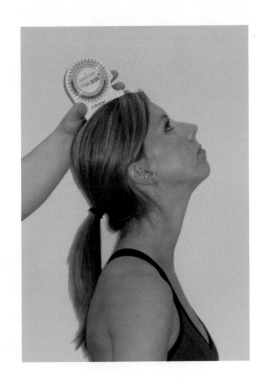

**Figure 5.6**
Cervical extension ROM with inclinometer.

## Intervention

Patients were treated for two sessions over 4–8 days. Treatment included:

- Manipulation: Three techniques repeated twice each
  - Seated distraction manipulation (**Figure 5.7**)
    - The patient was in a sitting position. The clinician placed his or her upper chest at the level of the patient's middle thoracic spine and grasped the patient's elbows. A high-velocity distraction thrust was performed in an upward direction.
  - Supine upper-thoracic spine manipulation (**Figures 5.8 and 5.9**)
    - The patient was in the supine position with his or her hands clasped across the base of the neck. The clinician used his or her manipulative hand to stabilize the inferior vertebra of the motion segment, targeted between T1 and T4, and used his or her body to push down through the subject's arms to perform a high-velocity, low-amplitude thrust.

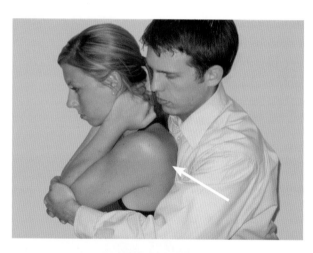

**Figure 5.7**
(Left) Seated distraction manipulation.

**Figure 5.8**
(Bottom left) Thoracic manipulation hand position.

**Figure 5.9**
(Bottom right) Supine upper-thoracic manipulation.

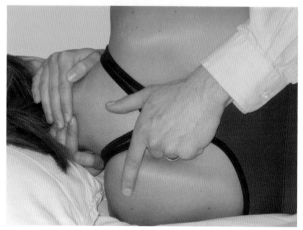

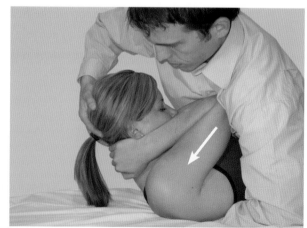

- Middle thoracic spine manipulation (**Figure 5.10**)
  - Identical to the upper-thoracic manipulation, except the patient grasped the opposite shoulder with his or her hands and the clinician targeted between T5 and T8 with the thrust.

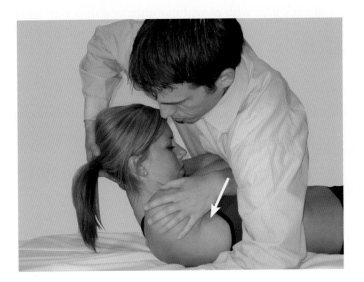

**Figure 5.10**
Supine mid-thoracic manipulation.

- Cervical ROM (**Figure 5.11**)
  - The patient placed his or her fingers over the manubrium and placed his or her chin on the fingers. The patient was instructed to rotate to one side as far as possible, and return to neutral.
  - Performed alternately to both sides within pain tolerance

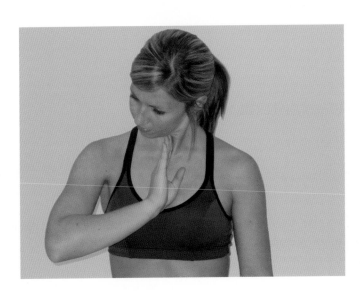

**Figure 5.11**
Cervical ROM exercise.

## Study Specifics

*Inclusion Criteria*

- Ages 18–60
- Primary complaint of neck pain with or without unilateral upper-extremity symptoms
- Baseline NDI score of ≥ 10%

*Exclusion Criteria*

- Identification of any medical "red flags" suggestive of a non-musculoskeletal etiology
- History of a whiplash injury within 6 weeks of the examination
- Diagnosis of cervical spinal stenosis
- Evidence of any central nervous system involvement
- Signs consistent with nerve root compression
  - At least two of the following diminished
    - Myotomal strength
    - Sensation
    - Reflexes

*Patient Characteristics*

- N = 78 subjects
- Mean age = 42.0 (+/– 11.3)
- Percentage of subjects considered a treatment success = 54%
- Mean duration of symptoms: 80 days (+/– 70.6)
- Gender
  - Female = 68%
  - Male = 42%

*Definition of Success*

- ≥ +5 (quite a bit better) on the GROC score

*Validation/Impact Analysis*

- None reported to date

## References

1. Cleland JA, Childs JD, Fritz JM, Whitman JM, Eberhart SL. Development of a clinical prediction rule for guiding treatment of a subgroup of patients with neck pain: use of thoracic spine manipulation, exercise, and patient education. *Phys Ther.* 2007;87:9–23.

## INTERVENTIONAL

# Treatment of Trigger Points for Chronic Tension-Type Headache[1]

## Predictor Variables

- Predictors of short-term success (1 week)
  1. Headache duration 8.5 hours per day
  2. Headache frequency < 5.5 days per week
  3. Bodily pain < 47
     a. From the SF-36
  4. Vitality < 47.5
     a. From the SF-36
- Predictors of long-term success (4 weeks)
  1. Headache frequency < 5.5 days per week
  2. Bodily pain < 47
     a. From the SF-36

## Clinical Bottom Line

The possession of two or more predictor variables indicates a small (4 weeks after discharge) to moderate (1 week after discharge) shift in probability that patients will receive a moderate perceived global improvement or a 50% decrease in headache frequency, intensity, or duration after 3 weeks of trigger-point therapy and exercise. The methodological quality of the derivation study was acceptable; therefore, it is appropriate to use this CPR as a component of the best available evidence.

## Intervention

Patients were treated for six sessions over 3 weeks. Treatment included:
- Trigger-point therapy
  - Focused on head, neck, and shoulder muscles
  - Temporalis, suboccipital, upper trapezius, superior oblique, splenius capitis, sternocleidomastoid, semispinalis capitis
  - Techniques included pressure release, muscle energy, soft tissue
- Home exercise program based on cervical extensors and deep neck flexors
  - Low-load and progressive contractions, 10 repetitions daily
  - Instruction to increase repetitions once patients achieve good control

**Interventional**

**Level: IV**

**Quality Score: 67%**

Short-Term Success

Trigger Point Therapy Indicated if:

**Two or More** Predictor Variables Present

**+LR 5.9**
(95% CI 0.8–42.9)

Long-Term Success

Trigger Point Therapy Indicated if:

**BOTH** Predictor Variables Present

**+LR 4.6**
(95% CI 1.2–17.9)

## Study Specifics

### Inclusion Criteria

- Pain characteristics of tension-type headache
  - Bilateral location
  - Pressing and tightening pain
  - Mild or moderate intensity ($\leq$ 6 on a 10 cm visual analogue scale)
  - No aggravation of pain during physical activity
- No reported photophobia, phonophobia, vomiting, or nausea during attacks
- Headaches for at least 15 days per month for last 3 months
- No evidence of secondary headache

### Exclusion Criteria

- Medication-overuse headache
- Pain features of migraine or other headache
- Identification of any medical "red flags"
- History of a whiplash injury
- History of cervical or cranial surgery
- Evidence of any central nervous system involvement

### Patient Characteristics

- N = 35 subjects
- Mean age = 39.7 (+/− 15.6)
- Percentage of subjects considered a treatment success = 55%
- Gender
  - Female = 77%
  - Male = 23%

### Definition of Success

- Headache diary
  - 50% reduction in at least one of the headache features
    - Headache intensity, frequency, or duration
- $\geq$ +5 (quite a bit better) on the GROC score

### Validation/Impact Analysis

- None reported to date

## References

1. Fernandez-de-las-Penas C, Cleland JA, Cuadrado ML, Pareja JA. Predictor variables for identifying patients with chronic tension-type headache who are likely to achieve short-term success with muscle trigger point therapy. *Cephalalgia*. 2008;28:264–275.

INTERVENTIONAL

# Cervical Traction for Mechanical Neck Pain[1]

## Predictor Variables

**1.** Age ≥ 55
**2.** Positive shoulder abduction test
**3.** Positive upper-limb tension test A (ULTT A)
**4.** Symptoms peripheralize with central posterior to anterior motion testing at C4–C7
**5.** Positive neck distraction test

| | |
|---|---|
| **Interventional** | |
| **Level: IV** | |
| **Quality Score: 67%** | |

Cervical Traction Indicated if:

**Three or More** Predictor Variables Present

**+LR 4.8** (95% CI 2.2–11.4)

## Clinical Bottom Line

The presence of three or more predictor variables creates a moderate shift in probability that an individual with neck pain will experience a large change or better in perceived benefit from mechanical cervical traction and exercise after 3 weeks. The methodological quality of the derivation study was acceptable; therefore, it is appropriate to use this CPR as a component of the best available evidence.

## Examination

- Positive shoulder abduction test (**Figure 5.12**)
  - The patient was asked to place the hand of the affected upper extremity on top of his or her head. The test was considered positive if his or her symptoms decreased.

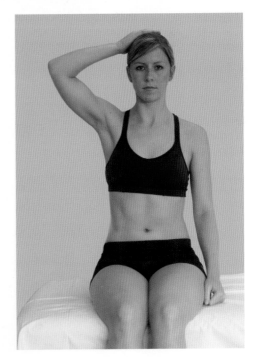

**Figure 5.12**
Shoulder abduction test.

- Positive upper-limb tension test A (ULTT A) (**Figure 5.13**)
    - ▪ Step 1          Scapular depression
    - ▪ Step 2          Shoulder abduction
    - ▪ Step 3          Forearm supination, wrist and finger extension
    - ▪ Step 4          Shoulder lateral rotation
    - ▪ Step 5          Elbow extension
    - ▪ Step 6A        Contralateral cervical side bending
    - ▪ Step 6B        Ipsilateral cervical side bending
- Positive if the patient's symptoms were reproduced, a side-to-side difference of > 10° in elbow extension was noted, or symptoms increased in Step 6A or decreased in Step 6B.

**Figure 5.13**
Upper-limb tension test A.

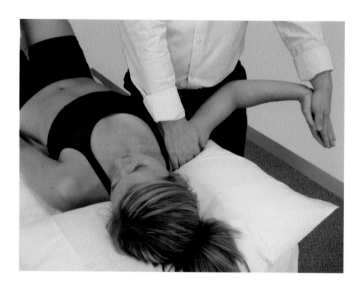

**Figure 5.14**
Central posterior-to-anterior motion testing at C4–C7.

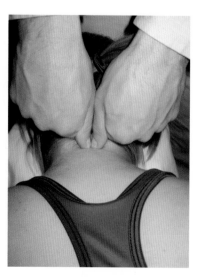

- Symptoms peripheralize with central posterior-to-anterior motion testing at C4–C7 (**Figure 5.14**)
    - ▪ The patient was in a prone position. The clinician located the spinous processes of C4–C7. The thumbs were used to apply a graded, oscillating mobilization to each spinous process. The variable was considered positive if any level caused symptoms to travel farther down the arm.

- Positive neck distraction test (**Figure 5.15**)
  - The patient was in a supine position. The clinician grasped the chin and occiput, flexed the patient's neck to a position of comfort, and gradually applied a distraction force up to ~14 kg. The test was considered positive if the patient's symptoms decreased.

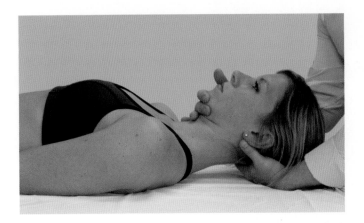

**Figure 5.15**
Neck distraction test.

## Intervention

Patients were treated for two to three sessions per week over 3 weeks, for a total of six sessions. Treatment included:

- Cervical traction (**Figure 5.16**)
  - Performed in a supine position with intermittent traction performed at an angle of 24° of flexion. The angle was adjusted to 15° if full cervical flexion wasn't possible. The traction was on for 60 seconds and off for 20 seconds. Fifty percent of pull was maintained during the off phase. Traction was initially set at 10–12 pounds and was increased to attempt to reduce symptoms. Traction time was 15 minutes.

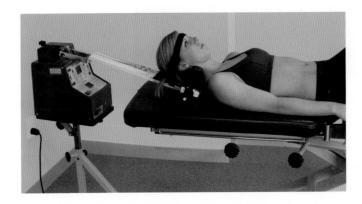

**Figure 5.16**
Cervical mechanical traction.

*Source:* Courtesy of the Chattanooga Group.

- Exercise
  - A seated posture exercise included retracting and adducting the scapula while elongating the cervical spine. The hold time was 10 seconds, and it was repeated for two repetitions per hour (**Figure 5.17**)

**Figure 5.17**
Seated upright posture.

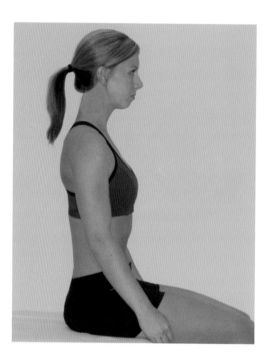

  - Supine deep-neck flexor strengthening performed via a craniocervical motion without contracting the large, superficial muscles. The contraction was held for 10 seconds and was repeated 10 times, twice per day (**Figure 5.18**)

**Figure 5.18**
Deep-neck flexor strengthening— capital rotation only.

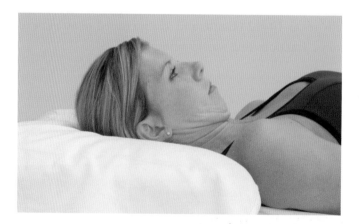

- Instruction to maintain normal activity without pain exacerbation

## Study Specifics

### Inclusion Criteria

- Ages ≥ 18
- Neck pain with or without upper-extremity symptoms
- Baseline NDI score of ≥ 20%

### Exclusion Criteria

- Red flags suggestive of a non-musculoskeletal etiology
- Pregnancy
- Evidence of vascular compromise
- Central nervous system involvement or multiple-level neurological impairments

### Patient Characteristics

- N = 68 subjects
- Mean age = 47.8 (+/− 7.2)
- Percentage of patients defined as a treatment success = 44%
- Mean duration of symptoms (days) = 292.4
- Gender
  - Female = 56%
  - Male = 44%

### Definition of Success

- ≥ +6 (a great deal better) on the GROC score

### Validation/Impact Analysis

- None reported to date

## References

1. Raney NH, Petersen EJ, Smith TA, et al. Development of a clinical prediction rule to identify patients with neck pain likely to benefit from cervical traction and exercise. *Eur Spine J.* 2009;18:382–391.

INTERVENTIONAL

# Prediction of Benefit or No Benefit with Occlusal Splint for Temporomandibular (TMJ) Pain[1]

| Interventional |
| :---: |
| **Level: IV** |
| **Quality Score: 72%** |

Occlusal Splint
Indicated if:

**All Four** Predictor
Variables Are Present

**+LR 10.8**
(95% CI 0.6–188.1)

Occlusal Splint **Not**
Indicated if:

**All Four** Non-Success
Predictors Present

**–LR 0.1**
(95% CI 0.0–0.8)

## Predictor Variables

1. Time since pain onset ≤ 42 weeks
2. Baseline visual analogue scale pain level ≥ 40 mm
3. Change in visual analogue scale level at 2-month follow-up ≥ 15 mm
4. Disc displacement without reduction

## Significant Predictor Variables of Failure

1. Time since pain onset > 43 weeks
2. Baseline visual analogue scale pain level < 22 mm
3. Change in visual analogue scale level at 2-month follow-up < 9 mm
4. Disc displacement with reduction

## Clinical Bottom Line

Individuals with persistent, unilateral TMJ arthralgia and all four variables predictive of success have a moderate shift in probability that they will experience improvements in pain at a 6-month follow-up. A large shift in the probability that an individual will not experience improvement in pain was also predicted by the presence of all four variables for failure. The methodological quality of the derivation study was acceptable; therefore, it is appropriate to use this CPR as a component of the best available evidence.

## Intervention

Patients were issued a hard-acrylic, full-arch maxillary stabilization-type splint with flat occlusal surfaces. The splint was used only at night and was used for 6 months.

## Study Specifics

*Inclusion Criteria*

- Unilateral TMJ diagnosis of arthralgia (per the Research Diagnostic Criteria for temporomandibular disorders)[2]

- > 2 months since pain onset
- Pretreatment visual analogue scale (VAS) pain level of > 10 mm
- Ages 18–70
- Ambulatory and able to be treated as an outpatient
- Available for study schedule

## Exclusion Criteria

- Pain attributable to confirmed migraine or head or neck pain condition
- Acute infection or other significant disease of the teeth, ears, eyes, nose, or throat
- Debilitating physical or mental illness
- Presence of a collagen vascular disease
- History of trauma
- History of temporomandibular disorder (TMD) treatment or joint surgery
- Inability to speak or write German

## Patient Characteristics

- N = 119 subjects
- Mean age = 34.6
- Percentage of subjects considered a treatment success = 55%
- Percentage of subjects considered a treatment failure = 14%
- Gender
  - Female = 92%
  - Male = 8%

## Definition of Success

- VAS change of 70% at the 6-month follow-up

## Definition of Failure

- VAS change of < 7 mm associated with baseline VAS levels of ≤ 40 mm
- VAS change of < 21 mm associated with baseline VAS levels of 40 mm to 70 mm
- VAS change of < 28 mm associated with baseline VAS levels of 70 mm to 100 mm

## Validation/Impact Analysis

- None reported to date

## References

1. Emshoff R, Rudisch A. Likelihood ratio methodology to identify predictors of treatment outcome in temporomandibular joint arthralgia patients. *Oral Surg Oral Med Oral Pathol Oral Radiol Endod.* 2008;106:525–533.
2. Dworkin SF, LeResche L. Research diagnostic criteria for temporomandibular disorders. Review, criteria, examinations, and specifications, critique. *J Craniomandib Disord.* 1992;6:301–355.

# UPPER EXTREMITIES

DIAGNOSTIC

# Diagnosis of Subacromial Impingement Syndrome and Full-Thickness Rotator Cuff Tear in Patient with Shoulder Pain[1]

| Diagnostic |
| --- |
| Level: IV |
| Impingement Syndrome if: |
| **All Three** Impingement Variables Present |
| **+LR 10.6** |
| Rotator Cuff Tear if: |
| **All Three Rotator** Cuff Tear Variables Present |
| **+LR 15.6** |

## Predictor Variables for Impingement Syndrome

**1.** Positive Hawkins–Kennedy impingement sign
**2.** Positive painful arc sign
**3.** Positive infraspinatus muscle strength test

## Predictor Variables for Full-Thickness Rotator Cuff Tear

**1.** Positive painful arc sign
**2.** Positive infraspinatus muscle test
**3.** Positive drop arm sign

## Clinical Bottom Line

This study provides clinicians with two test clusters to determine the probability that patients will have impingement syndrome or isolated full-thickness rotator cuff tear as diagnosed by arthroscopy. A large and conclusive shift in posttest probability is produced by the presence of three predictor tests. A methodological quality analysis is suggested before implementing this CPR as a component of the best available evidence.

## Examination

- Positive Hawkins-Kennedy (**Figure 6.1**)
  - The patient's arm was passively placed in a 90° forward flexion position, and then gently rotated into internal rotation. The test was considered positive if the patient felt pain.

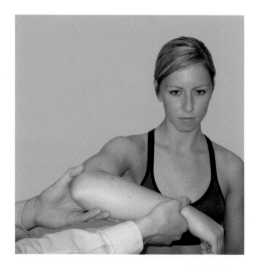

Figure 6.1
Hawkins–Kennedy test.

- Positive painful arc (**Figure 6.2**)
  - ◼ The patient actively elevated the arm in the scapular plane until full elevation was reached, then brought down the arm. Pain or catching between 60° and 120° of elevation was considered a positive test.

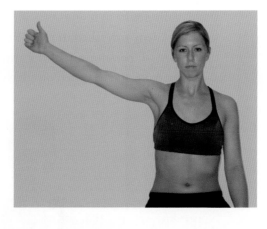

**Figure 6.2**
Painful arc test.

- Positive infraspinatus muscle test (**Figure 6.3**)
  - ◼ The patient's elbow was in 90° flexion with the shoulder in 0° abduction and neutral rotation. The clinician applied an internal rotation force to the arm while the patient resisted. The test was considered positive if the patient was unable to maintain external rotation because of weakness or pain, or if there was a positive external rotation lag sign. The external rotation lag sign was performed with the arm in same position; the clinician passively externally rotated the shoulder and the patient was asked to hold the position. If the patient could not maintain the rotated position, the test was considered positive.

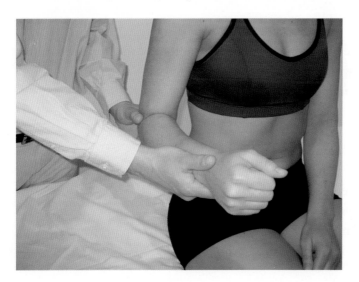

**Figure 6.3**
Infraspinatus muscle strength test.

- Positive drop arm sign (**Figure 6.4**)
  - ■ The patient was asked to elevate the arm fully, then to slowly reverse the motion in the same arc. If the arm dropped suddenly or the patient had severe pain, the test was considered to be positive.

**Figure 6.4**
Drop arm sign.

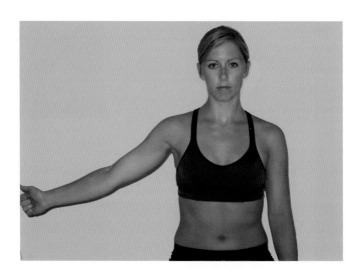

## Study Specifics

### Inclusion Criteria

- Patients who were examined by the senior author of the study with history
- Physical exam within 4 weeks of surgery
- Questionnaire entered into a database

### Exclusion Criteria

- History of shoulder surgery
- Acromioclavicular arthritis requiring excision of the distal part of the clavicle with impingement syndrome
- Incomplete physical examination due to limited motion or extreme pain
- Superior labrum anterior-to-posterior lesions with impingement syndrome
- Instability with impingement syndrome

### Patient Characteristics

- N = 359 subjects
- Prevalence of impingement but no rotator cuff disease = 20%
- Prevalence of full-thickness rotator cuff tears = 60%

*Definition of Positive (Reference Standard)*

- Diagnostic arthroscopy
  - Non-impingement group: normal rotator cuffs. May have a different pathologic condition such as instability, isolated degenerative acromio-clavicular arthritis, supraspinatus ganglion cyst, nonspecific synovitis, or superior labrum anterior-to-posterior lesion.
  - Impingement group: diagnosis on impingement syndrome regardless of severity. Subgrouped into three groups:
    - Positive impingement tests, but no rotator cuff disease at the time of surgery
    - Partial rotator cuff tear regardless of depth
    - Full-thickness rotator cuff tear, regardless of size
      - Including small tears, large tears, massive tears, or multiple tendon tears

*Validation/Impact Analysis*

- None reported to date

## References

1. Park HB, Yokota A, Gill HS, El Rassi G, McFarland EG. Diagnostic accuracy of clinical tests for the different degrees of subacromial impingement syndrome. *J Bone Joint Surg Am*. 2005;87:1446–1455.

DIAGNOSTIC

# Diagnosis of Rotator Cuff Tears[1]

**Diagnostic**

**Level: III**

Rotator Cuff Tear
Present if:

**Four or More** Total
Points

**+LR 9.8**

## Predictor Variables

|  | Score |
|---|---|
| **1.** Weakness on external rotation | 2 |
| **2.** Age ≥ 65 | 2 |
| **3.** Presence of night pain | 1 |

## Clinical Bottom Line

Individuals who score 4 or 5 points based on the identified three predictor variables have a moderate/large shift in probability that they possess a partial or large rotator cuff tear. This study has undergone internal validation confirming findings, indicating that more confidence can be used in application to clinical practice; however, caution in interpreting the results should be taken until broad validation is completed.

## Examination

- Weakness on external rotation (ER) (**Figure 6.5**)
  - The patient was positioned in sitting or standing position. The elbow was flexed to 90° and the shoulder was internally rotated 20°. The patient then resisted in the direction of ER. The test was considered positive if the therapist judged that weakness was present.

**Figure 6.5**
Testing weakness in external rotation.

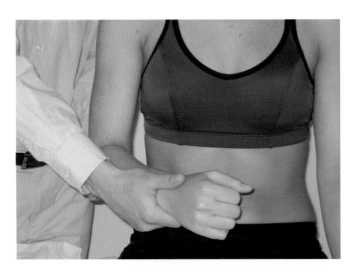

- Presence of night pain
  - Positive if the patient reported that he or she could not stay asleep due to shoulder pain

## Study Specifics

### Inclusion Criteria

- Status post arthrography for suspected rotator cuff tear

### Exclusion Criteria

- Arthrography was performed for suspected adhesive capsulitis
- Recent fracture involving the affected joint
- Recent operative procedure on the affected joint
- Radiographic evidence of osteoarthritis of the glenohumeral joint

### Patient Characteristics

- N = 448 subjects
- Mean age = 57.4 (+/− 12.6)
- Prevalence of a rotator cuff tear = 67.2%
- Gender
  - Female = 37%
  - Male = 63%

### Definition of Positive (Reference Standard)

- Evidence of partial or complete rotator cuff tear through contrast arthrography

### Validation

- Retrospective, internal validation of 216 subjects indicating a specificity of 91% to identify partial or complete rotator cuff tears at the cutoff score of 4+.[1] The quality score for this validation study was 40%.

## References

1. Litaker D, Pioro M, Bilbeisi HE, Brems J. Returning to the bedside: using the history and physical exam to identify rotator cuff tears. *J Am Geriatr Soc.* 2000;48:1633–1637.

DIAGNOSTIC

# Diagnosis of Carpal Tunnel Syndrome (CTS)[1]

| **Diagnostic** |
| --- |
| **Level: IV** |
| Diagnostic for CTS if: |
| **Four or More** Predictor Variables Present |
| **+LR 4.6** (95% CI 2.5–8.7) |

## Predictor Variables

1. Shaking hands relieves symptoms
2. Wrist-ratio index > 0.67
3. Brigham and Women's Hospital Hand Symptom Severity Scale (SSS) score > 1.9
4. Diminished sensation in median sensory field 1 (thumb)
5. Age > 45

## Clinical Bottom Line

The presence of four or more predictor variables indicates a small to moderate shift in probability that a patient will also test positive for CTS using needle electromyography (EMG). A methodological quality analysis is suggested before implementing this CPR as a component of the best available evidence.

## Examination

- Wrist-ratio index > 0.67
  - Anteroposterior (AP) and mediolateral (ML) wrist width was measured with sliding calipers in centimeters. The ratio was computed by dividing AP wrist width by ML wrist width.
- Brigham and Women's Hospital Hand SSS score > 1.9
  - SSS consists of 11 statement items related to six domains thought critical for the evaluation of CTS.
- Diminished sensation in median sensory field 1 (thumb)
  - Measured with pinprick and compared to the ipsilateral proximal aspect of the thenar eminence.

## Study Specifics

*Inclusion Criteria*

- Ages 18–70
- Recruited from primary care clinic, orthopedic department, and patients referred to the electrophysiologic laboratories of participating facilities
- Suspected cervical radiculopathy or CTS as judged by the electrophysiologic laboratory provider

## Exclusion Criteria

- Systemic disease known to cause a generalized peripheral neuropathy
- Primary complaint of bilateral radiating arm pain
- History of conditions involving the affected upper extremity that resulted in a reduced level of function
- Off work for > 6 months because of the condition
- History of surgical procedures for pathologies giving rise to neck pain or for CTS
- Previous needle EMG and nerve conduction study (NCS) testing of the symptomatic limb for cervical radiculopathy and/or CTS
- Subjects receiving workers' compensation or with pending litigation for their condition

## Patient Characteristics

- N = 82 subjects
- Mean age = 45 (+/− 12)
- Prevalence of CTS = 34%
- Gender
  - Female = 50%
  - Male = 50%

## Definition of Positive (Reference Standard)

- A diagnosis of a compatible clinical presentation and abnormal electrophysiologic findings as determined by a neurologist or physiatrist

## Validation/Impact Analysis

- None reported to date

## References

1. Wainner RS, Fritz JM, Irrgang JJ, Delitto A, Allison S, Boninger ML. Development of a clinical prediction rule for the diagnosis of carpal tunnel syndrome. *Arch Phys Med Rehabil.* 2005;86:609–618.

DIAGNOSTIC

# The American College of Rheumatology Criteria for the Classification of Osteoarthritis (OA) of the Hand[1]

| Diagnostic |
| --- |
| **Diagnostic** |
| **Level: III** |
| Diagnostic for OA of the Hand if: |
| **All Five** Predictor Variables Are Met |
| **+LR 46.0** |
| **−LR 0.1** |

## Predictor Variables

1. Hand pain, aching, or stiffness *and*
2. Hard tissue enlargement of two or more of 10 selected joints (distal interphalangeal (DIP) and proximal interphalangeal (PIP) joints of the second and third digits and the first carpometacarpal (CMC) joint of both hands) *and*
3. < 3 swollen metacarpophalangeal (MCP) joints *and either*
4. Hard tissue enlargement of two or more DIP joints *or*
5. Deformity of two or more of 10 selected joints

## Clinical Bottom Line

The presence of all five predictor variables creates a large and conclusive shift in probability that the patient will be diagnosed with hand OA by a panel of reviewers with access to lab and radiographic results, history, and physical exam findings. There is also a large shift in probability that patients who do not meet this rule will not have clinical OA. This rule has been validated and may be applied to practice within the confines of the study's parameters; however, further external, broad studies still need to be performed.

## Study Specifics

*Inclusion Criteria*

- Symptomatic and idiopathic hand OA
- Symptomatic non-OA hand pain as comparison group

*Exclusion Criteria*

- Secondary OA of the hand

*Patient Characteristics*

- N = 199 subjects
- 100 subjects with OA
  - 99 control subjects

- Mean age in the OA group = 64 (+/− 10)
  - Female = 71%
  - Male = 29%
- Mean age in the control group = 51 (+/− 15)
  - Female = 75%
  - Male = 25%

### Definition of Positive (Reference Standard)

- The reference standard was the clinical diagnosis of OA made by independent reviewers based upon the patient's history, physical examination findings, and radiographic features.

### Validation

- Internal cross validations were utilized by sequentially leaving out 10% of the data. Results indicated a Sn of 88% and a Sp of 93%.[1]

## References

1. Altman R, Alarcon G, Appelrouth D, et al. The American College of Rheumatology criteria for the classification and reporting of osteoarthritis of the hand. *Arthritis Rheum.* 1990;33:1601–1610.

PROGNOSTIC

# Prediction of Persistent Shoulder Pain[1]

**Prognostic**

**Level: III**

Prognostic Scoring
Charts

Calculating the Risk
of Persistent Shoulder
Pain at 6 Weeks and 6
Months

## Predictor Variables: Persistent Shoulder Symptoms at 6 Weeks

| Risk Factor | Score |
|---|---|
| Duration of complaints | |
| 6 weeks | 0 |
| 6–12 weeks | 7 |
| > 3 months | 11 |
| Gradual onset | 7 |
| Psychological complaints | 10 |
| Repetitive movements | 8 |
| Shoulder pain score (0–10) | *score* |
| Neck pain score at physical exam (0–18) | *score* |

| Score | Risk | Score | Risk |
|---|---|---|---|
| ≤ 2 | 20–30% | 17–21 | 60–70% |
| 3–7 | 30–40% | 22–27 | 70–80% |
| 8–11 | 40–50% | 28–36 | 80–90% |
| 12–16 | 50–60% | ≥ 37 | 90–100% |

## Predictor Variables: Persistent Shoulder Symptoms at 6 Months

| Risk Factor | Score |
|---|---|
| Duration of complaints | |
| 6 weeks | 0 |
| 6–12 weeks | 9 |
| > 3 months | 17 |
| Gradual onset | 10 |
| Concomitant low-back pain | 13 |
| Shoulder pain score (0–10) | *score* $\times$ *2* |
| Neck pain score at physical exam (0–18) | *score* |

| Score | Risk | Score | Risk |
|-------|------|-------|------|
| ≤ 1 | 10–20% | 40–49 | 50–60% |
| 2–16 | 20–30% | 50–61 | 60–70% |
| 17–28 | 30–40% | ≥ 62 | 70–100% |
| 29–39 | 40–50% | | |

## Clinical Bottom Line

This clinical prediction rule provides clinicians with a scoring system they can use to determine the percentage risk of the patient having persistent shoulder pain at 6 weeks. Given the findings of the validation study, the predictors of short-term disability may be appropriate for clinical use within the confines of the study's parameters.

## Examination

- Repetitive movements (at least 2 days per week): "Yes" or "No" answer per patient report
- Psychological complaints measured as part of the Tampa Scale of Kinesiophobia[2]
- Neck pain score: 0 = no pain; 3 = severe pain. Total pain scores for neck flexion, extension, side bending, rotation in neutral, rotation in flexion, and rotation in extension (0–18).

## Study Specifics

### Inclusion Criteria

- Ages ≥ 18
- Had not consulted their general practitioner (GP) or received any form of treatment for the afflicted shoulder in the preceding 3 months
- Sufficient knowledge of the Dutch language to complete questionnaires

### Exclusion Criteria

- Severe physical or psychological conditions
  - Fractures or luxation in the shoulder region
  - Rheumatic disease
  - Neoplasm
  - Neurological or vascular disorders
  - Dementia

*Patient Characteristics*

- N = 587 subjects
- Mean age = 51 (+/− 14)
- Subjects with persistent pain
  - 6 weeks = 70%
  - 6 months = 46%
- Gender
  - Female = 50%
  - Male = 50%

*Definition of Positive (Reference Standard)*

- Mailed questionnaire at 6 weeks, 3 months, and 6 months
  - Primary outcome measure: Patient perceived recovery measured on an 8-point scale
    - Patients who did not report full recovery or very much improvement were denoted as having "persistent symptoms"
  - Secondary outcome measures
    - Shoulder disability measured with 16-item shoulder disability questionnaire
    - Pain measured on 0–10 numerical rating scale
    - Severity of main complaint on a 0–10 numerical rating scale

*Validation/Impact Analysis*

- Prospective validation with a sample of 212 subjects comparing the discriminate ability of the originally derived rule in the validation population. They found that prediction of short-term disability (6 weeks) showed good discriminate ability. The predictors of long-term disability performed poorly, with only slightly better than chance ability to predict disability.[3]

## References

1. Kuijpers T, van der Windt DAWM, Boek AJP, et al. Clinical prediction rules for the prognosis of shoulder pain in general practice. *Pain*. 2006;120:276–285.
2. Kori SH, Miller RP, Todd DD. Kinesiophobia: a new view of chronic pain behavior. *Pain Manage*. 1990:35–43.
3. Kuijpers T, van der Heijden GJMG, Vergouwe Y, et al. Good generalizability of a prediction rule for prediction of persistent shoulder pain in the short term. *J Clin Epidemiol*. 2007;50:947–953.

## INTERVENTIONAL

# Mobilization with Movement (MWM) and Exercise for Lateral Epicondylalgia[1]

## Predictor Variables

**1.** Age < 49
**2.** Affected side pain free grip > 112 N (25 lbs)
**3.** Unaffected side pain free grip < 336 N (76 lbs)

## Clinical Bottom Line

The presence of two of the predictor variables creates a small but sometimes clinically meaningful shift in probability that the individual with lateral epicondylalgia will feel improved, much improved, or completely recovered after 3 weeks of MWM, exercise, and a home exercise program. The probability of success increased to 100% when all three variables were present; however, the N was small (4 subjects), thus the current recommendation of two variables. The methodological quality of the derivation study was acceptable; therefore, it is appropriate to use this CPR as a component of the best available evidence.

| Interventional |
| --- |
| Level: IV |
| Quality Score: 67% |

| MWM Indicated if: |
| --- |
| **Two** Predictor Variables Present |
| **+LR 3.7** (95% CI 1.0–13.6) |

## Intervention

Patients were treated for five sessions over 3 weeks. Treatment included:

- MWM directed to the elbow:
  - Lateral glide of the elbow *or* a posteroanterior glide of the radiohumeral joint
    - Lateral glide (**Figure 6.6**)
      - The patient was supine with the arm supported in a position of elbow extension and forearm pronation. The clinician placed his or her stabilizing hand over the distal humerus above the lateral epicondyle. The gliding hand was placed on the medial side of the proximal forearm just below the joint line. The lateral glide was applied with the gliding hand from medial to lateral. The force was approximately

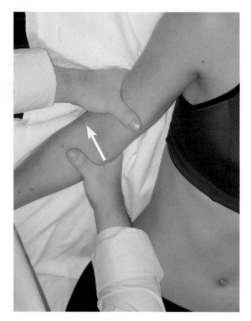

Figure 6.6
Lateral glide of the elbow.

two-thirds of the therapist's maximum force. The action, in this case gripping, should have decreased pain by ≥ 50%; if it did not, the angle of glide was adjusted from straight lateral to anterior lateral or slightly caudad until pain was relieved. Once the position was identified, the glide was maintained and the patient gripped (dynamometer for retest purposes) up to the onset of pain and no more. The grip was released followed by release of the glide. This was repeated 6–10 times.

- Posteroanterior glide of the radiohumeral joint (**Figure 6.7**)
  - If the lateral glide was ineffective, the posteroanterior glide was attempted. The starting position was the same with the stabilizing hand holding the distal humerus down on the table with the thumb over the radial head. The thumb of the other hand was placed on top of the stabilizing thumb while the hand rested on the forearm. The patient reproduced the aggravating activity while sustained PA pressure to the radial head was applied. If pain was reduced by ≥ 50%, the activity was repeated 6–10 times.

**Figure 6.7**
Posteroanterior glide of the radiohumeral joint.

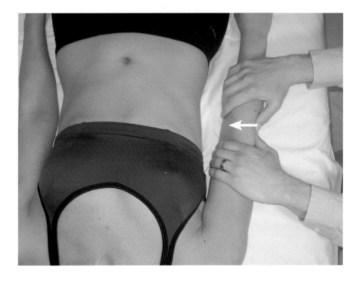

- Prescription of an exercise program to include home exercises and self-MWM:
  - Exercises
    - Including three sets of 8–12 repetitions with each repetition performed slowly lasting 6–10 seconds. Between sets 1–2 minutes was advised for proper rest. Examples included pain-free gripping with

exercise putty, resisted wrist extension, flexion, supination, pronation, ulnar, and radial deviation. Upper-quadrant muscle deficits were also addressed as needed to include modified bench presses with one arm, bent-over rows, unilateral shoulder press in the scapular plane, biceps curls, and triceps extensions in the supine position. Additionally, postural reeducation and work-simulated activities were issued as needed. Exercises were issued and progressed without creating pain either during or after the exercise.[2]

- Self-MWM
  - Self-lateral glides were performed by stabilizing the humerus either via a belt wrapped around the torso or the lateral arm propped up against the wall or door jam. The lateral glide was then applied with the unaffected hand, gliding medial to lateral until the activity (gripping, wrist extension, and so on) decreased pain. The activity was repeated 6–10 times (**Figures 6.8 and 6.9**)

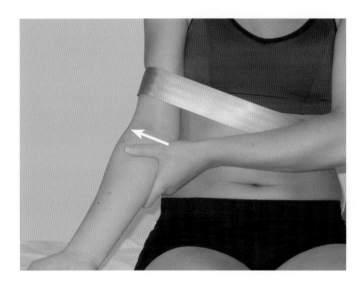

**Figure 6.8**
(Left) Self-lateral glide with belt.

**Figure 6.9**
(Below) Self-lateral glide against wall.

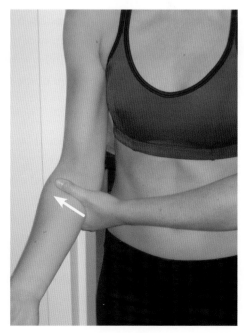

- Self-PA glides were performed in the supine position with the involved extremity internally rotated and pronated. The opposite noninvolved hand applied PA pressure via the middle and index finger until the activity pain was reduced (**Figure 6.10**)

**Figure 6.10**
Self-posteroanterior glide.

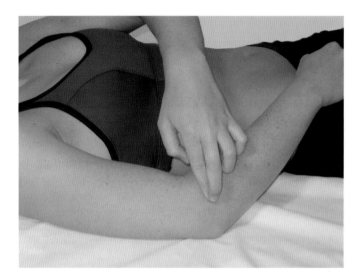

## Study Specifics

*Inclusion Criteria*

- Ages 18–65
- Pain over the lateral elbow of ≥ 6-weeks duration
- Pain is provoked by palpation of the lateral epicondyle, gripping, and extension of the wrist and second or third finger

*Exclusion Criteria*

- Treated by a health care practitioner for his or her lateral elbow pain in the preceding 6 months
- Bilateral elbow symptoms
- Cervical radiculopathy
- Concomitant shoulder, elbow, or hand pathology
- Peripheral nerve involvement
- Previous surgery of the elbow
- History of elbow dislocation, fracture, or tendon rupture
- Systemic neurological disorders
- Contraindications to steroids

*Patient Characteristics*

- N = 64 subjects
- Mean age = 48.2 (+/– 7.4)
- Percentage of subjects considered a treatment success = 79%
- Gender
  - Female = 34%
  - Male = 66%

*Definition of Success*

- Feeling "improved," "much improved," or "completely recovered" as per the 6-point Global Perceived Effect (GPE) scale.

*Validation/Impact Analysis*

- None reported to date

## References

1. Vicenzino B, Smith D, Cleland J, Bisset L. Development of a clinical prediction rule to identify initial responders to mobilization with movement and exercise for lateral epicondylalgia. *Man Ther.* 2009;14:550–554.
2. Vicenzino B. Lateral epicondylalgia: a musculoskeletal physiotherapy perspective. *Man Ther.* 2003;8:66–79.

INTERVENTIONAL

# Cervicothoracic Manipulation for Shoulder Pain[1]

**Interventional**

**Level: IV**

**Quality Score: 72%**

Cervicothoracic
Manipulation
Indicated if:

**Three or More**
Predictor Variables
Present

**+LR 5.3**
(95% CI 1.7–16.0)

## Predictor Variables

**1.** Pain free active shoulder flexion < 127°
**2.** Shoulder internal rotation < 53°
**3.** Negative Neer impingement test
**4.** Not taking any medication for the shoulder pain
**5.** Duration of symptoms < 90 days

## Clinical Bottom Line

The presence of three predictor variables creates a moderate shift in probability that the individual with shoulder pain will experience a moderate self-perceived global improvement, reduced shoulder disability, and improved active ROM from manual therapy and exercise, directed at the cervicothoracic spine, within two treatment sessions (4–8 days). The methodological quality of the derivation study was acceptable; therefore, it is appropriate to use this CPR as a component of the best available evidence.

## Examination

- Active shoulder flexion
  (**Figure 6.11**)
  - The patient was in the standing position and elevated his or her arm to the point of maximal, pain-free shoulder flexion. The fulcrum of the goniometer was placed close to the acromion process. The proximal arm was aligned with the midaxillary line of the trunk while the distal arm was aligned at the midline of the humerus.

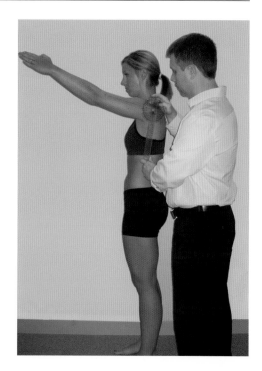

**Figure 6.11**
Active shoulder flexion.

- Shoulder internal rotation (**Figure 6.12**)
  - The patient was in the supine position. The arm was abducted to 90°, and a towel was placed under the distal humerus. The fulcrum was placed over the olecranon process with the proximal arm perpendicular to the floor and the distal arm in alignment with the ulna. The clinician then passively internally rotated the arm.

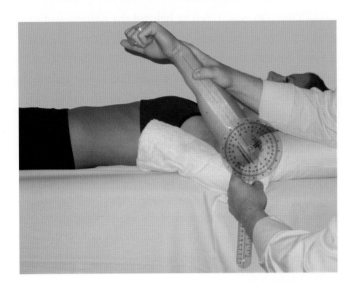

**Figure 6.12**
Shoulder internal rotation.

- Neer impingement test (**Figure 6.13**)
  - The patient was in the standing position. The clinician stabilized the scapula of the painful shoulder and forced the patients arm into maximal elevation. The test is positive if pain is produced.

**Figure 6.13**
Neer impingement test.

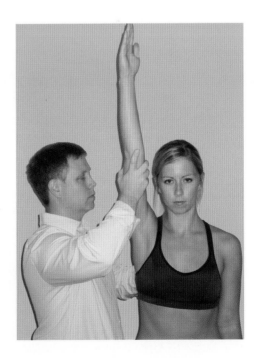

## Intervention

Patients were treated for one to two sessions over 4–8 days. Treatment included:

- Manual treatment: Thrust manipulations were performed twice, non-thrust manipulations were performed once
  - Middle thoracic spine distraction thrust manipulation (**Figure 6.14**)
    - The patient was in the sitting position with his or her arms crossed over the chest. The clinician was standing behind the patient and placed his or her hands around the trunk grasping the elbows. The clinician's chest or a towel roll was used as the fulcrum on the patient's middle thoracic spine. The high-velocity, low-amplitude thrust manipulation was applied in the posterior and slightly superior direction.
  - Lower cervical spine lateral translatory non-thrust manipulation (**Figure 6.15**)
    - The patient was in the hook-lying position. The clinician cradled the patients head with his or her index fingers contacting the postero-lateral region of the C5 vertebrae. A lateral translatory non-thrust manipulation (grade III and IV) was performed in both directions. The technique was repeated for 3 bouts of 30 seconds at each segment from C5–C7 and was performed in the cervical neutral as well as the cervical flexion position.

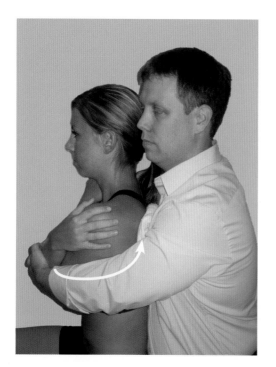

**Figure 6.14**
(Left) Middle thoracic spine distraction thrust manipulation.

**Figure 6.15**
(Below) Lower cervical spine lateral translatory non-thrust manipulation.

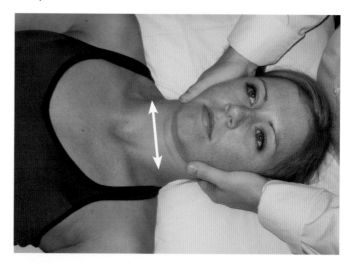

■ Cervicothoracic junction thrust manipulation (**Figure 6.16**)

  ● The patient was in the supine position. The patient's hands were clasped behind the base of the patient's neck. The clinician placed his or her hand at the cervicothoracic junction, stabilizing the T1 vertebrae. The patient's head and neck were flexed through the elbows down to the C7 level. The patient bridged upward to localize the effort. A high-velocity, low-amplitude thrust was applied through the patient's elbows from anterior to posterior.

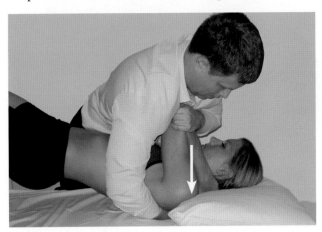

**Figure 6.16**
Cervicothoracic junction thrust manipulation.

■ Upper thoracic spine thrust manipulation (**Figure 6.17**)

  ● The patient was in the supine position with the hands clasped across the base of the neck. The clinician used his or her manipulative hand to stabilize the inferior vertebra of the motion segment, targeted between T1 and T4. A high-velocity, low-amplitude thrust was applied through the patient's elbows from anterior to posterior.

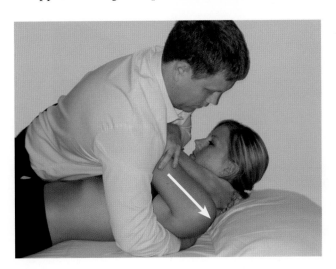

**Figure 6.17**
Upper thoracic spine thrust manipulation.

- Middle thoracic spine thrust manipulation (**Figure 6.18**)
  - Identical to the upper thoracic manipulation, except the patient grasped the opposite shoulder with his or her hands, and the clinician targeted between T5 and T8 with the thrust.

**Figure 6.18**
Middle thoracic spine thrust manipulation.

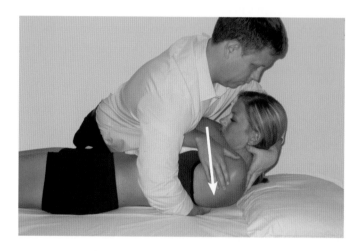

- Prone middle thoracic and lower thoracic spine thrust manipulation (**Figure 6.19**)
  - The patient was in the prone position with his or her arms by his or her sides. The clinician places his or her pisiforms on the transverse processes on each side of the identical vertebrae. A "skin lock" was achieved by rotating the hands slightly while pushing caudally with one hand and cranially with the other. The clinician applied a high-velocity, low-amplitude thrust through his or her extended arms from posterior to anterior.

**Figure 6.19**
Prone middle thoracic and lower thoracic thrust manipulation.

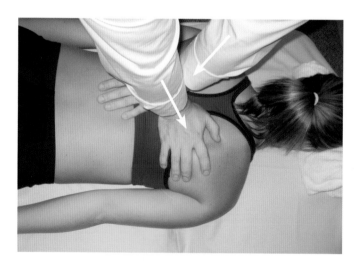

- Exercise: Each exercise was performed for 10 repetitions, 3–4 times per day
  - Three-finger AROM exercise (**Figure 6.20**)
    - The patient placed his or her stacked fingers above the manubrium and flexed the cervical spine down to that level. The patient was instructed to rotate to one side as far as possible and return to neutral. The motion was performed alternately to both sides within pain tolerance.

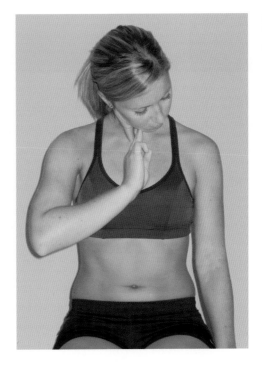

**Figure 6.20**
Three-finger AROM exercise.

  - Supine thoracic extension (**Figure 6.21**)
    - The patient was in the hook-lying position with a towel roll placed perpendicular to the spine. The patient placed his or her hands behind the neck and extended back using the towel roll as the fulcrum.

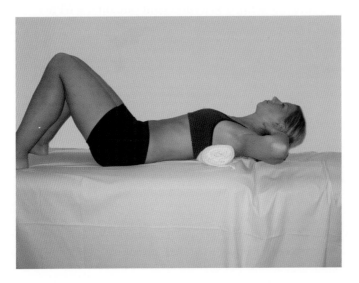

**Figure 6.21**
Supine thoracic extension.

  - Instructions to maintain pain free daily activities

## Study Specifics

*Inclusion Criteria*

- Ages 18–65
- Primary report of shoulder pain
- Baseline Shoulder Pain and Disability Index (SPADI) score of ≥ 20%

*Exclusion Criteria*

- Red flags suggesting a non-musculoskeletal cause of the patient's symptoms
- Acute fractures of the shoulder region
- Acute, severe trauma in the cervical or thoracic regions in the last 6 weeks
- Cervical spinal stenosis or bilateral upper extremity symptoms
- Osteoporosis
- Prior surgery to the cervical or thoracic regions
- Evidence of central nervous system involvement
- Signs of nerve root compression to include (2 or more of the following): myotomal strength changes, dermatomal sensations changes, reflex changes
- Insufficient English language skills to complete the required paperwork

*Patient Characteristics*

- N = 80 subjects
- Mean age = 40.4 (+/– 13.5)
- Percentage of subjects defined as a successful outcome = 61%
- Gender
  - Female = 59%
  - Male = 41%

*Definition of Success*

- ≥ +4 (moderately better) on the GROC score

*Validation/Impact Analysis*

- None reported to date

## References

1. Mintken PE, Cleland JA, Carpenter KJ, Bieniek ML, Keirns M, Whitman JM. Identifying prognostic factors for successful short-term outcomes in individuals with shoulder pain receiving cervicothoracic manipulation. *Phys Ther*. 2009;In Press.

# LUMBOPELVIC REGION

DIAGNOSTIC

# Diagnosis of Patients with Lumbar Spinal Stenosis (LSS)[1]

| | |
|---|---|
| **Diagnostic** | |
| **Level: III** | |
| Diagnosis of LSS if: | |
| **Seven or Higher** on Scoring System | |
| **+LR 3.9** | |
| LSS Likely Not Present if: | |
| **Two or Lower** on Scoring System | |
| **−LR 0.2** | |

## Predictor Variables

| | Score |
|---|---|
| **1.** Age | |
| 60–70 | 2 |
| > 70 | 3 |
| **2.** Symptoms present > 6 months | 1 |
| **3.** Symptoms improve when bending forward | 2 |
| **4.** Symptoms improve when bending backwards | −2 |
| **5.** Symptoms exacerbated while standing up | 2 |
| **6.** Intermittent claudication (+) (symptoms with walking; improve with rest) | 1 |
| **7.** Urinary incontinence (+) | 1 |

## Clinical Bottom Line

This rule can be used to help screen patients with lower-extremity symptoms for lumbar spinal stenosis as defined by an expert panel. A score of greater than seven indicates a small but perhaps meaningful shift in probability for LSS and a score of less than or equal to two produces a moderate shift in probability that the individual does not have LSS. This rule has been validated and may be applied to practice within the confines of the study parameters; however, further external, broad validation studies still need to be performed.

## Study Specifics

*Inclusion Criteria*

- Primary complaint of pain or numbness in the lower extremities, including the buttocks, thighs, and lower legs
- Ages > 20
- Able to visit the clinic alone without assistance

*Exclusion Criteria*

- Visited other hospitals or clinics in the past year for similar symptoms
- Severe psychiatric disorders

*Patient Characteristics*

- N = 468 subjects
- Mean age = 65.2 (+/− 13.7)
- Prevalence of lumbar spinal stenosis = 47.3%
- Gender
  - Female = 46%
  - Male = 54%

*Definition of Positive (Reference Standard)*

- Clinical and diagnostic test information including X-rays and MRIs were utilized via orthopedic specialists, the study coordinator, and a consensus panel to determine the diagnosis of lumbar spinal stenosis.

*Validation/Impact Analysis*

- Retrospective, internal validation of 94 Japanese patients indicating a likelihood ratio of 0.15 for individuals in the low-risk category, thus validating the ability of this rule to serve as a screening mechanism.[1]

## References

1. Sugioka T, Hayashino Y, Konno S, Kikuchi S, Fukuhara S. Predictive value of self-reported patient information for the identification of lumbar spinal stenosis. *Fam Pract*. 2008;25:237–244.

## DIAGNOSTIC

# Diagnosis of Pain Originating from the Sacroiliac Joint (SIJ)[1]

**Diagnostic**

**Level: IV**

Diagnostic of Pain from the SIJ if:

**Three or More** Predictor Variables Present

**+LR 4.3** (95% CI 2.3–8.6)

## Predictor Variables

For diagnosis of sacroiliac joint pain
1. Positive SIJ compression test
2. Positive SIJ distraction test
3. Positive femoral shear test
4. Positive sacral provocation
5. Positive right Gaenslen's test
6. Positive left Gaenslen's test

## Clinical Bottom Line

The presence of three or more predictor variables indicates a moderate shift in probability that a patient's back, buttock, and leg pain is arising from the SIJ when compared to diagnostic injection. A methodological quality analysis is suggested before implementing this CPR as a component of the best available evidence. Of note, the data analysis process did not use the common CRR techniques of regression analyses or recursive partitioning.

## Examination

For diagnosis of sacroiliac joint (SIJ) pain
- SI compression test (**Figure 7.1**)
  - The patient was in the left-side lying position and the clinician introduced a compressive force through the iliac crest. The test was considered positive if the patient's familiar symptoms were reproduced.
- SI distraction test (**Figure 7.2**)
  - The patient was in the supine position. The clinician placed the heel of his or her hand on the medial aspect of both anterior superior iliac spines (ASISs). A posterolateral force was applied through the right ASIS. The test was considered positive if the patient's familiar symptoms were reproduced.
- Femoral shear test (**Figure 7.3**)
  - The patient was in the supine position with the right hip and knee positioned in 90° flexion. The clinician introduced a posterior force through the femur. The test was considered positive if the patient's familiar symptoms were reproduced.

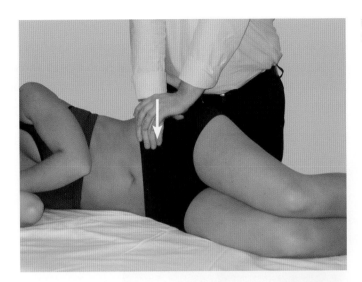

**Figure 7.1**
SI compression test.

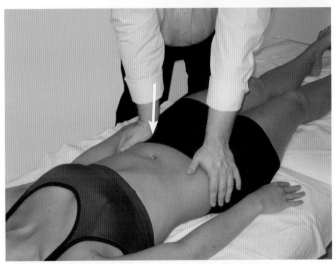

**Figure 7.2**
SI distraction test.

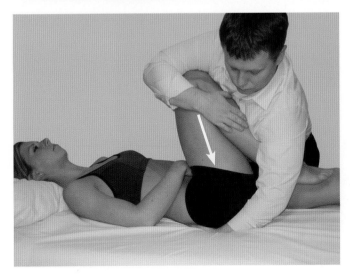

**Figure 7.3**
Femoral shear test.

- Sacral provocation (**Figure 7.4**)
  - The patient was in the prone position. The clinician placed the heel of his or her hand over the patient's sacrum and applied a posterior to anterior force. The test was considered positive if the patient's familiar symptoms were reproduced.

**Figure 7.4**
Sacral provocation test.

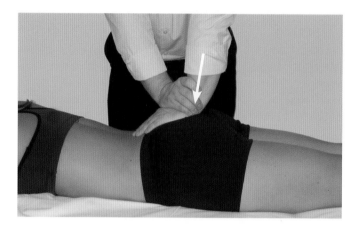

- Right Gaenslen's test (**Figure 7.5**)
  - The patient was in the supine position with the right leg over the edge of the treatment table and the left hip and knee held in flexion. The clinician placed his or her hand over the patient's right thigh and ASIS and introduced hip extension and anterior pelvic tilt while maintaining left-hip flexion. The test was considered positive if the patient's familiar symptoms were reproduced.
- Left Gaenslen's test
  - Same procedure as above repeated on the opposite side.

**Figure 7.5**
Gaenslen's test.

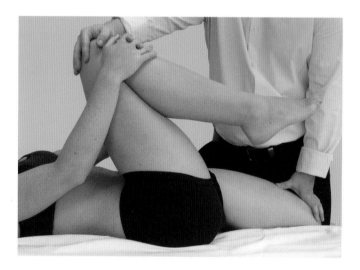

## Study Specifics

*Inclusion Criteria*

- Buttock pain with or without lumbar or lower-extremity symptoms
- Had undergone imaging and unsuccessful therapeutic interventions

*Exclusion Criteria*

- Unwilling to participate
- Midline or symmetrical pain above the level of L5
- Signs of nerve root compression
  - Complete motor or sensory deficit
- Referred for procedures excluding SIJ injection
- Patients deemed too frail to tolerate a full physical examination
- Pain free on the day of clinical assessment
- Bony obstruction leading to inability to perform injection

*Patient Characteristics*

- N = 48 subjects
- Mean age = 42.1 (+/− 12.3)
- Prevalence of patients with positive SIJ injections = 33%
- Mean symptom duration (months) = 31.8 (+/− 38.8)
- Gender
  - Female = 67%
  - Male = 33%

*Definition of Positive (Reference Standard)*

- Reference standard was fluoroscopy-guided SIJ injection
  - Injection test was positive if slow injection of solutions provoked familiar pain and injection of < 1.5 cc local anesthetic resulted in 80% or more relief from pain
  - Injection test was negative or indeterminate if there was no provocation of familiar pain, or if familiar pain was provoked, but there was insufficient pain relief

*Validation/Impact Analysis*

- None reported to date

## References

1. Laslett M, Aprill CN, McDonald B, Young SB. Diagnosis of sacroiliac joint pain: validity of individual provocation tests and composites of tests. *Man Ther*. 2005;10:207–218.

PROGNOSTIC

# Diagnosis of Ankylosing Spondylitis (AS)[1]

| Prognostic |
| --- |
| **Level: IV** |
| Diagnostic for Ankylosing Spondylitis if: |
| **Three or More** Predictor Variables Present |
| **+LR 12.4** (95% CI 4.0–39.7) |

## Predictor Variables

**1.** Morning stiffness > 30 minutes duration
**2.** Improvement in back pain with exercise but not with rest
**3.** Awakening because of back pain during the second half of the night only
**4.** Alternating buttock pain

## Clinical Bottom Line

The presence of three or more predictor variables indicates a large shift in probability that a patient's chronic low back pain is due to ankylosing spondylitis. A methodological analysis is suggested before implementing this CPR as a component of the best available evidence.

## Study Specifics

*Inclusion Criteria*

- Ages ≤ 50
- Chronic low back pain lasting ≥ 3 months
- Diagnosis of AS by rheumatologist or other specialist

*Patient Characteristics*

- N = 101 patients with AS
- Mean duration of back pain (years) = 12.9 (+/– 8.6)
- Mean age = 35.9 (+/– 7.9)
- Gender
  - Female = 36%
  - Male = 64%
- Comparison group of 112 subjects with mechanical low back pain

*Definition of Positive (Reference Standard)*

- Satisfaction of the modified New York criteria
  - Low back pain (improved with exercise, not relieved by rest)
  - Limited lumbar motion
  - Reduced chest expansion

- Bilateral grade > 2 sacroilitis on X-ray
- Unilateral grade 3 or 4 sacroilitis on X-ray

*Validation/Impact Analysis*

- None reported to date

## References

1. Rudwaleit M, Metter A, Listing J, Sieper J, Braun J. Inflammatory back pain in ankylosing spondylitis. *Arthritis Rheum*. 2006;54:569–578.

PROGNOSTIC

# Prediction of Recovery in Patients with Low Back Pain (LBP)[1]

**Prognostic**

**Level: III**

Recovery Likely if:

**All Three** Predictor Variables Present

**60%** Recovered at 1 week

**95%** Recovered at 12 weeks

## Predictor Variables

1. Baseline pain ≤ 7/10
2. Duration of current episode ≤ 5 days
3. Number of previous episodes ≤ 1

## Clinical Bottom Line

The presence of all three predictor variables identified individuals receiving spinal manual therapy and diclofenac who would be 95% recovered at 12 weeks, where recovery was defined as 0–1 out of 10 pain for 7 consecutive days. This rule has been validated and may be applied to practice within the confines of the study's parameters; however, further external, broad studies still need to be performed.

## Intervention

The study was a secondary analysis of a randomized controlled trial involving diclofenac and spinal manipulative therapy (95% non-thrust, 6% thrust). Treatment groups were

- Placebo spinal manipulative therapy and placebo diclofenac
- Placebo spinal manipulative therapy and active diclofenac
- Active spinal manipulative therapy and placebo diclofenac
- Active spinal manipulative therapy and active diclofenac

## Study Specifics

*Inclusion Criteria*

- Consecutive patients with low back pain, with or without leg pain
  - LBP defined as pain between the 12th rib and the buttock crease
- Presenting to 1 of 40 general practitioners
- Less than 6 weeks duration
- Moderate pain and disability
  - Measured by adaptations of items 7 and 8 of the SF-36

## Exclusion Criteria

- Current episode not preceded by a pain-free period of at least 1 month without care
- Known or suspected serious spinal pathology
- Nerve root compression
  - Determined by the presence of two or more of the following
    - Myotomal weakness
    - Dermatomal sensory loss
    - Hyporeflexia
- Currently receiving nonsteroidal anti-inflammatory drugs
- Currently receiving spinal manipulative therapy
- Surgery within the preceding 6 months
- Contraindication to paracetamol, diclofenac, or spinal manipulative therapy

## Patient Characteristics

- N = 239 subjects
- Mean age = 40.7 (+/− 15.6)
- Gender
  - Female = 44%
  - Male = 56%

## Definition of Success

- Recovery was defined as 7 days of 0 or 1 pain on a scale of 0–10

## Validation/Impact Analysis

- Internal validation within the same study comparing the prediction rule with therapist judgment. Results found that the prediction rule performed better then therapist judgment in predicting recovery.[1]

## References

1. Hancock MJ, Maher CG, Latimer J, Herbert RD, McAuley JH. Can rate of recovery be predicted in patients with acute low back pain? Development of a clinical prediction rule. *Eur J Pain*. 2009;13:51–55.

## INTERVENTIONAL

# Lumbar Stabilization for Low Back Pain[1]

**Therapeutic**

**Level: IV**

**Quality Score:
72%—Success Rule**

**67%—Failure Rule**

Success with
Stabilization Likely if:

**Three or More**
Predictor Variables of
Success Present

**+LR 4.0**
(95% CI 1.6–10.0)

Failure with
Stabilization Likely if:

**Three or More**
Predictor Variables of
Nonsuccess Present

**–LR 0.2**
(95% CI 0.2–0.4)

### Predictor Variables of Success

1. Straight leg raise (SLR) > 91°
2. < 40 years old
3. Aberrant motion present with forward bending
4. Positive prone instability test

### Predictor Variables of Nonsuccess

1. Fear Avoidance Belief Questionnaire—Physical activity < 8
2. Aberrant movement absent
3. No hypermobility during posterior to anterior (P-A) spring testing
4. Negative prone instability test

### Clinical Bottom Line

The presence of at least three success predictor variables indicates a small but sometimes meaningful increase in the probability that the patient will experience at least a 50% improvement in function after 8 weeks of lumbar stabilization. The presence of at least two of the nonsuccess predictor variables indicates a moderate shift in probability that the patient will not improve with lumbar stabilization. The methodological quality of the derivation study was acceptable; therefore, it is appropriate to use this CPR as a component of the best available evidence.

### Examination

- SLR > 91° (**Figure 7.6**)
  - The patient was in a supine position. An inclinometer was positioned on the tibial crest just below the tibial tubercle. The clinician lifted the patient's leg, keeping the knee straight. The measurement was taken at maximum tolerated SLR height, not at the onset of pain.
- Aberrant motion with forward bending
  - Noted with standing lumbar ROM, including instability catch, painful arc of motion, thigh climbing (Gower's sign) (**Figure 7.7**), or a reversal of lumbopelvic rhythm.

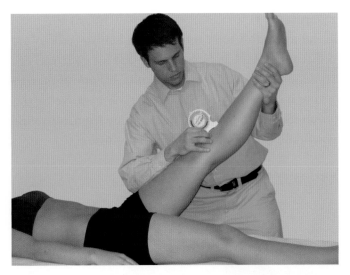

**Figure 7.6**
Straight leg raise with inclinometer.

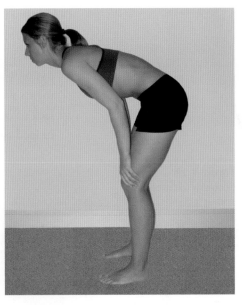

**Figure 7.7**
Aberrent motion—Gower's sign.

- Positive prone instability test
  - The patient was in a prone position with his or her body on the examining table and his or her legs over the edge and feet on the floor. In this position, the clinician applied posterior to anterior pressure to the lumbar spine (**Figure 7.8**). The patient was asked to report provocation of pain. If pain was reported, the patient lifted his or her legs off the floor (the patient could hold the table to maintain position) and P-A pressure was repeated at the same segment (**Figure 7.9**). If pain was present in the resting position, but subsided in the second position, the test was considered positive. The test was considered negative if there was no pain on initial spring testing, or if pain did not change or increase with lifting of the legs.

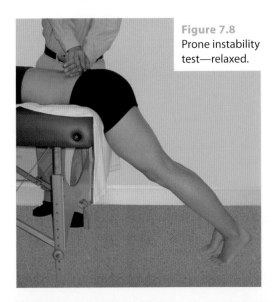

**Figure 7.8**
Prone instability test—relaxed.

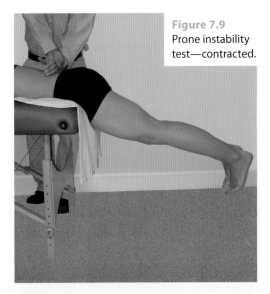

**Figure 7.9**
Prone instability test—contracted.

- P-A spring testing (**Figure 7.10**)
  - The clinician introduced a P-A force through each lumbar spinous process using his or her pisiform. A judgment was made for each level of hypomobile, hypermobile, or within normal limits. If none of the segments were noted to be hypermobile, the variable was negative for the lack of benefit from stabilization CPR. If one or more segments were judged to be hypermobile, then the variable was positive.

**Figure 7.10**
Posterior to anterior spring test.

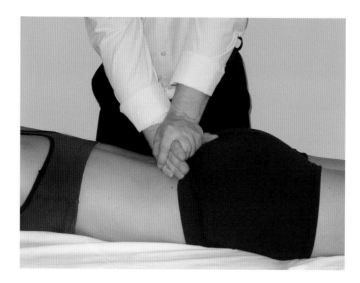

## Intervention

Patients were treated two times per week for 8 weeks. Treatment included:
- Exercise
  - Focus on rectus abdominus, transversus abdominus, internal oblique abdominals, erector spinae, multifidus, and quadratus lumborum

## Study Specifics

### Inclusion Criteria

- LBP with or without leg pain
- Ages > 18

### Exclusion Criteria

- Previous spinal fusion surgery
- LBP attributable to current pregnancy
- Acute fracture, tumor, or infection

- Presence of two or more of the following signs of nerve root compression
  - Diminished lower-extremity strength
  - Diminished lower-extremity sensation
  - Diminished lower-extremity reflexes

*Patient Characteristics*

- N = 54 subjects
- Mean age 42.2 (+/– 12.7)
- Percentage of patients defined as a treatment success = 33%
- Gender
  - Female = 57%
  - Male = 43%

*Definition of Success*

- > 50% improvement on the modified Oswestry Disability Index (ODI)
- Nonsuccess defined as a < 6 point improvement on the modified ODI

*Validation/Impact Analysis*

- None reported to date

## References

1. Hicks GE, Fritz JM, Delitto A, McGill SM. Preliminary development of a clinical prediction rule for determining which patients with low back pain will respond to a stabilization exercise program. *Arch Phys Med Rehabil.* 2005;86:1735–1762.

INTERVENTIONAL

# Lumbar Manipulation for Acute Low Back Pain (Success)[1]

**Interventional**

**Level: II**

Lumbar Manipulation
Indicated if:

**Four or More**
Predictor Variables
Present

**+LR 24.4**
(95% CI 4.6–139.4)

## Predictor Variables

**1.** Pain does not travel below the knee
**2.** Onset ≤ 16 days ago
**3.** Lumbar hypomobility
**4.** Either hip has > 35° of internal rotation
**5.** Fear Avoidance Belief Questionnaire—Work subscale score < 19

## Clinical Bottom Line

The presence of four or more predictor variables creates a large and conclusive shift in probability that the acute low back pain individual will experience at least a 50% improvement in function from lumbopelvic manipulation and exercise within two treatment sessions (4–8 days). This rule has been validated and may be applied to practice within the confines of the study's parameters.

## Examination

- Lumbar hypomobility (**Figure 7.11**)
  - The patient was in the prone position. The clinician introduced a P-A force through each lumbar spinous process using his or her pisiform. A judgment was made for each level of hypomobile, hypermobile, or within normal limits. If one or more segments were judged to be hypomobile, the variable was positive. If no segments were judged to be hypomobile, the variable was negative.

**Figure 7.11**
Lumbar hypomobility.

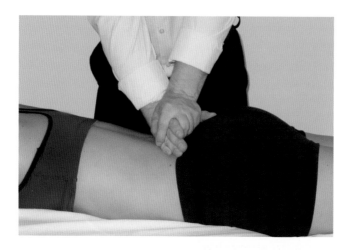

- Either hip has > 35° of internal rotation (**Figure 7.12**)
  - The patient was in the prone position. The involved leg was in line with the body with the knee flexed to 90°, while the contralateral leg was slightly abducted. The inclinometer was placed just inferior to the lateral malleolus. The hip was passively internally rotated until the contralateral pelvis began to rise, and the measurement was taken.

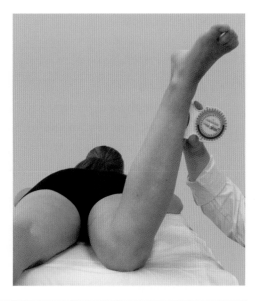

**Figure 7.12**
Hip internal rotation ROM with inclinometer.

## Intervention

Patients were treated for one to two sessions over 4–8 days. Treatment included:

- Lumbopelvic manipulation (**Figure 7.13**)
  - The clinician stood opposite the side to be manipulated. The patient was passively side bent away from the therapist. The clinician passively rotated the patient and then delivered a quick posterior and inferior thrust through the anterior superior iliac spine. If a cavitation was heard, the therapist proceeded to the other treatment components. If no cavitation was heard, the patient was repositioned and manipulated again. If no cavitation was heard on the second attempt, the opposite side was attempted for a maximum of two times per side.

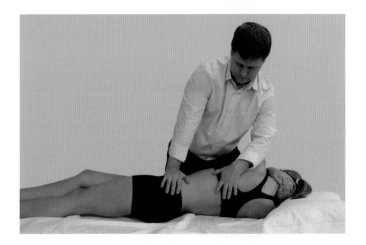

**Figure 7.13**
Lumbopelvic manipulation.

- Supine pelvic tilt home exercise program
- Instruction to maintain usual activity levels within limits of pain

## Study Specifics

*Inclusion Criteria*

- Ages 18–60
- Referral to physical therapy with a diagnosis related to the lumbosacral spine
- Chief complaint of pain and/or numbness in the lumbar spine, buttock, and/or lower extremity
- Modified Oswestry Disability Index score ≥ 30%

*Exclusion Criteria*

- Pregnancy
- Signs consistent with nerve root compression
  - Positive SLR at < 45°, or diminished lower-extremity strength, sensation, or reflexes
- Prior lumbar spine surgery
- History of osteoporosis
- History of spinal fracture

*Patient Characteristics*

- N = 71 subjects
- Mean age = 37.6 (+/– 10.6)
- Percentage of patients defined as a treatment success = 45%
- Gender
  - Female = 41%
  - Male = 59%

*Definition of Success*

- > 50% improvement on the modified ODI

*Validation/Impact Analysis*

- Prospective broad validation randomizing groups into exercise-only and manipulation groups. Patients' outcome at 1 and 4 weeks, and 6 months were assessed in relation to their status on the CPR. Those patients who were positive on the CPR and received manipulation had odds of success of 60.8 (95% CI 5.2–704.7) and less utilization of health care resources at 6 months. The number needed to treat for benefit at 4 weeks was 19.0 (95% CI 1.4–3.5).[2] The quality score for this validation study was 50%.

- Secondary analysis of two studies[1,2] found that using only 2 prognostic variables, duration less than 16 days and no symptoms below the knee, was predictive of patients who would benefit from manipulation (positive LR 7.1).[3]
- Secondary analysis of a randomized controlled trial[4] comparing patient status on the clinical prediction rule to outcomes at 1, 2, 4, and 12 weeks. All patients received advice and paracetemol from their general practitioner. They were randomized to a control group: placebo manipulation and placebo diclofenac or placebo manipulation and active diclofenac; or to a manipulation group: active manipulation and placebo diclofenac, or active manipulation and active diclofenac. Manipulative therapy included both low-velocity oscillatory (97%) and high-velocity, low-amplitude (5%) procedures. Results indicated that the rule did not generalize to individuals receiving primarily low-grade manipulative procedures.[5] The quality score for this validation study was 50%.

## References

1. Flynn T, Fritz J, Whitman J, et al. A clinical prediction rule for classifying patients with low back pain who demonstrate short-term improvement with spinal manipulation. *Spine*. 2002;27:2835–2843.
2. Childs JD, Fritz JM, Flynn TW, et al. A clinical prediction rule to identify patients with low back pain most likely to benefit from spinal manipulation: a validation study. *Ann Intern Med*. 2004;141:920–928.
3. Fritz JM, Childs JD, Flynn TW. Pragmatic application of a clinical prediction rule in primary care to identify patients with low back pain with a good prognosis following a brief spinal manipulation intervention. *BMC Fam Pract*. 2005;6:29.
4. Hancock MJ, Maher CG, Latimer J, Herbert RD, McAuley JH. Addition of diclofenac and/or manipulation to advice and paracetamol does not speed recovery from acute low back pain: a randomized controlled trial. *Lancet*. 2007;370:1638–1643.
5. Hancock MJ, Maher CG, Latimer J, Herbert RD, McAuley JH. Independent evaluation of a clinical prediction rule for spinal manipulative therapy: a randomized controlled trial. *Eur Spine J*. 2008;17:936–943.

INTERVENTIONAL

# Lumbar Manipulation for Acute Low Back Pain (Failure)[1]

Interventional

Level: IV

Quality Score: 61%

## Significant Predictor Variables Independently Associated with Failure

| | Odds Ratio (95% CI) |
|---|---|
| Decreased average total hip rotation ROM | 0.95 (0.90–1.00) |
| Longer duration of symptoms | 1.03 (1.01–1.06) |
| Not having low back pain only | 0.14 (0.01–1.46) |
| Negative Gaenslen's test | 0.11 (0.02–0.68) |
| Absence of lumbar hypomobility (spring test) | 0.09 (0.01–0.84) |
| Decreased hip medial rotation ROM discrepancy between sides | 0.68 (0.51–0.90) |

## Clinical Bottom Line

The variables included in this prediction rule help to identify which individuals may not improve by ≥ 5 points on the modified ODI, after lumbar manipulation and range of motion exercises over two treatment sessions. The methodological quality of the derivation study was acceptable; therefore, it is appropriate to use this CPR as a component of the best available evidence.

## Examination

- Gaenslen's test (**Figure 7.14**)
  - The patient was in the supine position with the leg of the side to be tested over the edge of the treatment table and the contralateral hip and knee held in flexion by the patient's arms. The clinician placed his or her hand over the patient's thigh and ASIS and introduced hip extension and anterior pelvic tilt. The test was considered positive if the patient's familiar symptoms were reproduced.

**Figure 7.14**
Gaenslen's test.

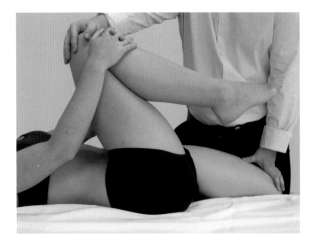

- Lumbar hypomobility (**Figure 7.15**)
  - The patient was in the prone position. The clinician introduced a posterior to anterior force through each lumbar spinous process using his or her pisiform. A judgment was made for each level of hypomobile, hypermobile, or within normal limits.

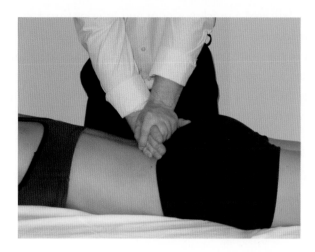

**Figure 7.15**
Posterior to anterior spring test.

- Hip internal rotation ROM (**Figure 7.16**)
  - The patient was in the prone position. The patient's involved leg was in line with the body with the knee flexed to 90°, while the contralateral leg was slightly abducted. The inclinometer was placed just inferior to the lateral malleolus. The hip was passively internally rotated until the contralateral pelvis began to rise, and the measurement was taken. The measurements between the right and left side were compared.

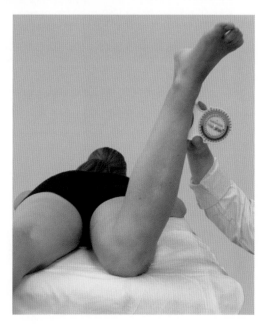

**Figure 7.16**
Hip internal rotation ROM with inclinometer.

## Intervention

Patients were treated for one to two sessions over 4–8 days. Treatment included:

- Lumbopelvic manipulation (**Figure 7.17**)
  - The clinician stood opposite the side to be manipulated. The patient was passively side bent away from the therapist. The clinician passively rotated the patient and then delivered a quick posterior and inferior thrust through the anterior superior iliac spine. If a cavitation was heard, the therapist proceeded to the other treatment components. If no cavitation was heard, the patient was repositioned and manipulated again. If no cavitation was heard on the second attempt, the opposite side was attempted for a maximum of two times per side.

**Figure 7.17** Lumbopelvic manipulation.

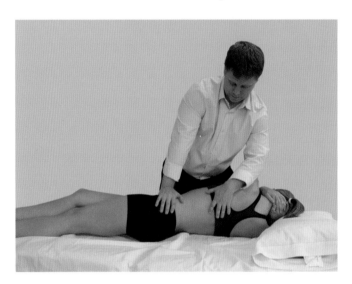

- Supine pelvic tilt home exercise program
- Instruction to maintain usual activity levels within limits of pain

## Study Specifics

### Inclusion Criteria

- Ages 18–60
- Referral to physical therapy with a diagnosis related to the lumbosacral spine
- Chief complaint of pain and/or numbness in the lumbar spine, buttocks, and/or lower extremity
- Modified Oswestry Disability Questionnaire score of ≥ 30%

*Exclusion Criteria*

- Pregnancy
- Signs consistent with nerve root compression
  - Positive straight-leg raise at < 45°, or diminished lower-extremity strength, sensation, or reflexes
- Prior lumbar spine surgery
- History of osteoporosis
- History of spinal fracture

*Patient Characteristics*

- N = 71 subjects
- Mean age = 37.6 (+/− 10.6)
- Percentage of patients defined as a treatment nonsuccess = 28%
- Gender
  - Female = 41%
  - Male = 59%

*Definition of a Lack of Success*

- Improvement on the Oswestry Disability Questionnaire of ≤ 5 points

*Validation/Impact Analysis*

- None reported to date

## References

1. Fritz JM, Whitman JM, Flynn TW, Wainner RS, Childs JD. Factors related to the inability of individuals with low back pain to improve with a spinal manipulation. *Phys Ther*. 2004;84:173–190.

INTERVENTIONAL

# Prone Lumbar Mechanical Traction in Patients with Signs of Nerve Root Compression[1]

**Interventional**

**Level: IV**

**Quality Score: 61%**

Prone Mechanical Traction Indicated if:

**Either** Predictor Variable Present

Differentiated **84%** with Recovery Using Traction vs

Only **45%** with Recovery without Traction

### Predictor Variables

**1.** Peripheralization with repeated lumbar extension
**2.** Positive crossed SLR

### Clinical Bottom Line

The presence of one or more predictor variable helps to identify patients with signs of nerve root compression who have a higher likelihood of experiencing a 50% reduction in disability after 6 weeks of manual therapy, extension exercises, lumbar traction, and education. The methodological quality of the derivation study was acceptable; therefore, it is appropriate to use this CPR as a component of the best available evidence.

### Examination

- Peripheralization with repeated lumbar extension (**Figure 7.18**)
  - Standing, the patient repeatedly bent backward for 10 repetitions to assess the change in lower extremity symptoms. If symptoms moved distally it was considered peripheralizaton.

**Figure 7.18**
Repeated extension in standing.

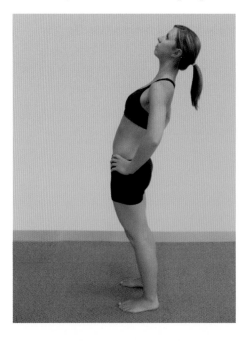

- Positive crossed straight leg raise (**Figure 7.19**)
  - The patient was in the supine position. The clinician passively elevated the straight leg on the contralateral side. The test was considered positive if contralateral symptoms were reproduced.

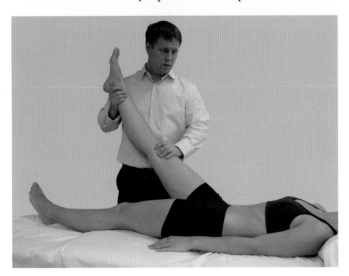

**Figure 7.19**
Crossed straight leg test.

## Intervention

Patients were treated for a maximum of 12 sessions over 6 weeks. Treatment included:

- Mechanical traction (**Figure 7.20**)
  - An adjustable table was used allowing for flexion/extension, rotation, or side-bending modifications. The patient was in the prone position with table adjusted to maximize centralization. Static traction at 40–60% body-weight for a maximum of 12 minutes was applied. If the table was not initially in the extension position, the table was repositioned after 3 minutes of traction in a more tolerable position, with the goal of reaching neutral or extended spine. The patient remained prone for 2 minutes after completing traction, then performed 10 prone press-ups prior to standing up.
  - Only used during the first 2 weeks of treatment.

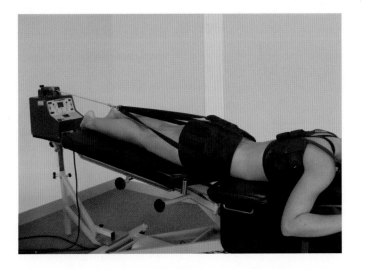

**Figure 7.20**
Prone lumbar traction.
*Source:* Courtesy of the Cattanooga Group.

- Extension exercises
  - Sustained and repeated lumbar extension in the prone and standing positions
  - Exercises were progressed as tolerated with emphasis on achieving maximum extension ROM without peripheralization
  - Three sets of 10 exercises throughout the day every 4–5 hours
- Manual therapy
  - Grade 3 or 4 oscillation of posterior to anterior mobilization
    - PT selected grade and spinal level
- Education
  - Maintain the lumbar lordosis while sitting
  - Discontinuation of any activities that caused peripheralization of symptoms

## Study Specifics

### Inclusion Criteria

- Ages 18–60
- Symptoms of pain and/or numbness extending distal to the buttock in the past 24 hours
- Modified Oswestry Disability Index score ≥ 30%
- Signs of nerve root compression
  - Positive SLR with reproduction of symptoms at < 45°
  - Reflex, sensory, or muscle strength deficit

### Exclusion Criteria

- Medical red flags indicative of nonmechanical LBP
- Previous spinal fusion or spine surgery in the past 6 months
- Current pregnancy
- Absence of any symptoms while sitting

### Patient Characteristics

- N = 64 subjects
  - 49 subjects included in traction CPR analysis
- Mean age = 41.1 (+/− 9.8)
- Total population percentage of subjects considered a treatment success = 60.9%
- Median symptom duration (days) = 47.5

- Gender
  - Female = 56%
  - Male = 44%

*Definition of Success*

- Modified Oswestry Disability Index change of ≥ 50%

*Validation/Impact Analysis*

- None reported to date

## References

1. Fritz JM, Lindsay W, Matheson JW, et al. Is there a subgroup of patients with low back pain likely to benefit from mechanical traction? *Spine*. 2007;32:E793–E800.

INTERVENTIONAL

# Supine Lumbar Mechanical Traction for Low Back Pain[1]

Interventional

Level: IV

Quality Score: 72%

Mechanical Traction
Indicated if:

**All Four** Predictor
Variables Present

**+LR 9.4**
(95% CI 3.1–28.0)

## Predictor Variables

1. Fear Avoidance Belief Questionnaire—Work subscale < 21
2. No neurological deficits
3. > 30 years old
4. Nonmanual work job status

## Clinical Bottom Line

The presence of all four predictor variables helps to identify patients with LBP that have a higher likelihood of experiencing a 50% reduction in disability after three sessions of intermittent, mechanical lumbar traction in supine. The methodological quality of the derivation study was acceptable; therefore, it is appropriate to use this CPR as a component of the best available evidence.

## Intervention

Patients were treated for three sessions over 9 days. Treatment included:

- Mechanical traction (**Figure 7.21**)
  - Patient was in the supine position with the hips and knees supported and flexed to 90°. A straight supine position was used for individuals who could not tolerate the hip and knee flexed position; 30–40% of body weight traction was applied. An intermittent approach was used with a 30-second hold and a 10-second relaxation phase for 15 minutes.
- Advice to stay active

**Figure 7.21**
Supine traction with knees and hips at 90°.
*Source:* Courtesy of the Cattanooga Group.

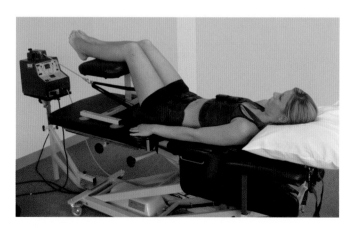

## Study Specifics

*Inclusion Criteria*

- Diagnosis with lumbosacral spine involvement
- Chief complaint of pain and/or numbness in the lumbar spine, buttock, and/or lower extremity

*Exclusion Criteria*

- Current pregnancy
- Signs of spinal cord injury
- Prior lumbar spine surgery
- Osteoporosis
- Spinal fracture

*Patient Characteristics*

- N = 129 subjects
- Mean age = 30.9 (+/− 12)
- Percentage of subjects considered a treatment success = 19.4%
- Gender
  - Female = 16%
  - Male = 84%

*Definition of Success*

- Modified Oswestry Disability Index change of > 50%

*Validation/Impact Analysis*

- None reported to date

## References

1. Cai C, Pua YH, Lim KC. A clinical prediction rule for classifying patients with low back pain who demonstrate short-term improvement with mechanical lumbar traction. *Eur Spine J.* 2009;18:554–561.

INTERVENTIONAL

# Facet Joint Block in Low Back Pain[1]

**Interventional**

**Level: IV**

**Quality Score: 56%**

Facet Joint Block Indicated if:

**Four or More**
Predictor Variables Present

**+LR 7.6**
(95% CI 4.5–13.7)

**Less Than Four**
Predictor Variables Present

**–LR 0.0**
(95% CI 0.0–0.5)

## Predictor Variables

1. Age ≥ 50
2. Symptoms best with walking
3. Symptoms best with sitting
4. Onset pain is paraspinal
5. Positive extension rotation test
6. Modified Somatic Perception Questionnaire[2] > 13
7. Absence of centralization

## Clinical Bottom Line

The study identifies a CPR with a strong ability to rule out patients likely not to experience a 75–95% decrease in pain lasting at least 1.5 hours from facet joint blocks. It also identifies a rule with moderate ability to identify patients likely to benefit from diagnostic facet blocks. The methodological quality of this study is below the suggested standard, so results should be taken with caution if this CPR is used clinically before validation.

## Examination

- Positive extension rotation test (**Figure 7.22**)
  - The patient was standing, and actively side bent, extended, and rotated toward the painful side. This could be achieved by instructing the patient to slide his or her ipsilateral hand down the back of the ipsilateral thigh. The variable was positive if pain was reproduced.

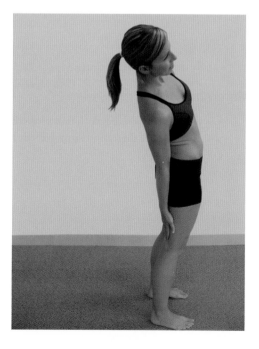

**Figure 7.22**
Extension rotation test.

## Study Specifics

### Inclusion Criteria

- Low back pain with or without lower extremity symptoms

### Exclusion Criteria

- Too frail to undergo the physical examination
- Inability to comprehend the study procedures

### Patient Characteristics

- N = 120 subjects
- Mean age = 43 (+/− 13)
- Percentage of patients defined as a treatment success (75% VAS reduction) = 24.2%
- Percentage of patients defined as a treatment success (95% VAS reduction) = 10.8%
- Mean duration of pain (weeks) = 158 (+/− 184)

### Definition of Success

- Greater than 75% or 95% (two analyses performed) Visual Analogue Scale (VAS) pain reduction after facet joint or medial branch diagnostic blocks lasting ≥ 1.5 hours depending on the anesthetic.

### Validation/Impact Analysis

- None reported to date

## References

1. Laslett M, McDonald B, Aprill CN, Trop H, Oberg B. Clinical predictors of screening lumbar zygapophyseal joint blocks: development of clinical prediction rules. *Spine J*. 2006;6:370–379.
2. Main CJ. The modified somatic pain questionnaire (MSPQ). *J Pscychosom Res*. 1983;27:503–514.

INTERVENTIONAL

# Response to Exercise in Ankylosing Spondylitis (AS)[1]

**Interventional**

**Level: IV**

**Quality Score: 72%**

Exercise Indicated if:

**Two or More** Predictor Variables Present

**+LR 11.2**
(95% CI 1.7–76.0)

## Predictor Variables

1. Bath Ankylosing Spondylitis Disease Activity Index > 31
2. SF-36: Role limitations due to physical problems > 37
3. SF-36: Bodily pain > 27

## Clinical Bottom Line

The presence of two or more predictor variables creates a large and conclusive shift in probability that the patient with AS will likely experience moderate perceived global improvement or improved functioning from an exercise program dispensed over 15 treatment sessions. The methodological quality of the derivation study was acceptable; therefore, it is appropriate to use this CPR as a component of the best available evidence.

## Intervention

Subjects were treated for 15 one-hour sessions over 15 weeks. Treatment included:
- General warm-up: two sets of eight repeats each
  - Stretching exercises of the posterior and anterior muscle chain
  - Neural mobilization of the median nerve
- Specific warm-up: two series of eight repeats each
  - A-P pelvic girdle gliding
  - McKenzie extensions
  - Stretching of the anterior and posterior pelvic musculature
- Dynamic axial exercise: two series of 10 each
  - Prone anterior pelvic girdle gliding
  - Supine A-P pelvic girdle gliding
  - Rotational stretching of the posterior musculature
- Static postural exercise: sustained 3–4-minute holds each
  - Supine anterior muscle chain stretches
  - Seated anterior and posterior muscle chain stretches
  - Standing anterior muscle chain stretching
  - Eccentric erector spine muscles

- Specific respiratory exercises: two series of 10 repeats each
  - Thoracic breathless
  - Expiratory breathless
  - Stretching of the anterointernal muscle chain of the scapular girdle
- Cooling down: one series of five repeats each
  - Cervical flexoextension
  - Cervical lateral-flexion
  - Cervical rotation
  - Circular motion of the scapular girdle

## Study Specifics

### Inclusion Criteria

- Diagnosis of AS as per the modified New York criteria

### Exclusion Criteria

- Medical condition that impaired function more than AS
- Osteoporosis or history of fracture due to osteoporosis
- Presence of symptoms from any other concomitant chronic disease

### Patient Characteristics

- N = 35 subjects
- Mean age: 45.7 (+/– 8.7)
- Percentage of patients defined as a treatment success = 46%
- Mean duration of symptoms (years) = 9.7 (+/– 2.6)
- Gender
  - Female = 20%
  - Male = 80%

### Definition of Success

- ≥ +5 (quite a bit better) on the GROC score *or*
- ≥ 20% improvement Bath Ankylosing Spondylitis Functional Index

### Validation/Impact Analysis

- None reported to date

## References

1. Alonso-Blanco C, Fernandez-de-las-Penas C, Cleland JA. Preliminary clinical prediction rule for identifying patients with ankylosing spondylitis who are likely to respond to an exercise program: a pilot study. *Am J Phys Med Rehabil*. 2009;88:445–454.

# LOWER EXTREMITIES

DIAGNOSTIC

# The American College of Rheumatology Criteria for the Classification of Osteoarthritis (OA) of the Hip[1]

| Diagnostic |
| --- |
| **Level: III** |
| Hip Osteoarthritis Present if: |
| **All** Variables From **Either** Cluster Are Present |
| **+LR 3.4** |
| **–LR 0.2** |

## Predictor Variables

**Cluster 1**
- Hip pain
- Hip internal rotation < 15°
- Hip flexion ≤ 115°

**Cluster 2**
- Hip pain
- Hip internal rotation ≥ 15°
- Pain on hip internal rotation
- Hip morning stiffness ≤ 60 minutes
- > 50 years old

## Clinical Bottom Line

There is a small but sometimes important shift in probability that patients with hip pain who meet all criteria from either of the above clusters will have clinical OA as compared to a diagnosis made by a clinician with access to all history, physical, radiograph, and lab results. There is also a moderate shift in probability that patients who do not meet either cluster do not have clinical OA. This rule has been validated and may be applied to practice within the confines of the study's parameters; however, further external, broad studies still need to be performed.

## Examination

- Hip internal rotation < 15°
  - Measurement technique not reported
  - Recommended technique (**Figure 8.1**)
    - Patient in the prone position with the knee flexed to 90°. The inclinometer is zeroed on the wall and then placed just inferior to the lateral malleolus. The hip is brought into internal rotation until the contralateral pelvis begins to rise and the measurement is taken.

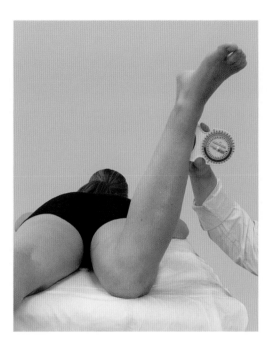

**Figure 8.1**
Hip internal rotation ROM with inclinometer.

- Hip flexion ≤ 115°
  - ▪ Measurement technique not reported
  - ▪ Recommended technique (**Figure 8.2**)
    - The patient is in the supine position. The axis of a goniometer is placed at the greater trochanter, the stationary arm is in line with the midaxillary line, and the moving arm is in line with the femur pointing at the lateral femoral epicondyle. The examiner passively flexes the hip maximally and the measurement is taken when the opposite thigh begins to rise off of the table.

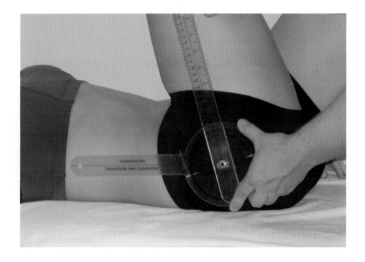

**Figure 8.2**
Hip flexion ROM with goniometer.

## Study Specifics

*Inclusion Criteria*

- Symptomatic hip OA
- Hip pain due to causes other than hip OA were enrolled as a comparison group

*Exclusion Criteria*

- None described

*Patient Characteristics*

- N = 201 subjects
- 114 subjects with hip OA
  - 87 control subjects
- Mean age in the OA group = 64 (+/− 13)
  - Female = 43%
  - Male = 57%
- Mean age in the control group = 57 (+/− 15)
  - Female = 28%
  - Male = 72%

*Definition of Positive (Reference Standard)*

- Diagnosis of hip OA by the contributing center using all available tests, measures, history, lab, and radiographic information
  - Diagnosis was independently reviewed by a subcommittee for verification of the diagnosis

*Validation/Impact Analysis*

- Internal cross validations were utilized by sequentially leaving out 10% of the data. Results indicated a Sn of 83% and a Sp of 68%.[1]

## References

1. Altman R, Alarcon G, Appelrouth D, et al. The American college of rheumatology criteria for the classification and reporting of osteoarthritis of the hip. *Arthritis Rheum*. 1991;34:505–514.

DIAGNOSTIC

# Diagnosis of Hip Osteoarthritis (OA)[1]

## Predictor Variables

1. Squatting as an aggravating factor (self-reported)
2. Active hip flexion causes lateral hip pain
3. Scour test with adduction causes lateral hip or groin pain
4. Active hip extension causes pain
5. Passive internal rotation of ≤ 25°

## Clinical Bottom Line

Patients who present with three or more predictor variables have at least a moderate shift in probability that they will have radiographic signs of hip OA. A methodological analysis is suggested before implementing this CPR as a component of the best available evidence.

**Diagnostic**

**Level: IV**

Diagnostic for Hip Osteoarthritis if:

**Three or More** Predictor Variables Present

**+LR 5.2**
(95% CI 2.6–10.9)

## Examination

- Active hip flexion (**Figure 8.3**)
  - The patient was in the supine position with knee extended. He or she was asked to actively flex the hip. The test was positive if lateral hip pain was reproduced.
- Active hip extension (**Figure 8.4**)
  - The patient was in the prone position with knee extended. He or she was asked to actively extend the hip. The test was positive if pain was reproduced.

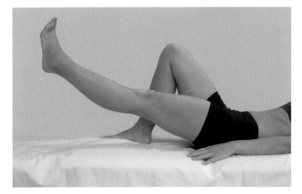

**Figure 8.3**
Active hip flexion.

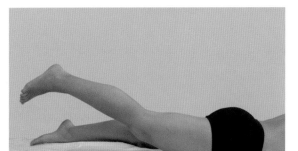

**Figure 8.4**
Active hip extension.

- Passive internal rotation of ≤ 25° (**Figure 8.5**)
    - ▪ The patient was in the prone position. The involved leg was in line with the body with the knee flexed to 90°, and the contralateral leg was slightly abducted. The inclinometer was placed just inferior to the lateral malleolus. The hip was passively internally rotated until the contralateral pelvis began to rise, and the measurement was taken.
- Scour test (**Figure 8.6**)
    - ▪ The patient was in the supine position with the hip flexed to 90°. The clinician passively moved the femur toward the opposite shoulder and axial pressure was applied downward toward the hip. If groin pain was not reproduced, hip internal rotation and adduction with axial pressure were added to further test the area. This variable was considered positive if groin pain was reproduced with the addition of adduction and axial pressure.

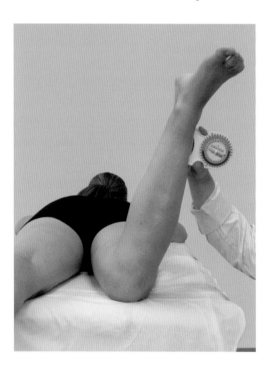

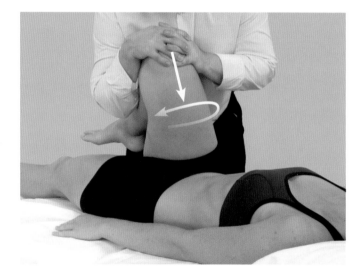

**Figure 8.5**
(Below, left) Hip internal rotation ROM with inclinometer.
**Figure 8.6**
(Below, right) Scour test with adduction.

## Study Specifics

*Inclusion Criteria*

- Ages > 40
- Primary complaint of unilateral pain in the buttock, groin, or anterior thigh

## Exclusion Criteria

- Current diagnosis or cancer
- History of hip surgery
- Pregnant females at the time of the study

## Patient Characteristics

- N = 72 subjects
- Mean age = 58.6 (+/− 11.2)
- Prevalence of subjects diagnosed with hip OA = 29%
- Gender
  - Female = 56%
  - Male = 44%

## Definition of Positive (Reference Standard)

- A Kellgren–Lawrence score of ≥ 2 on radiographs was considered positive for hip OA

## Validation/Impact Analysis

- None reported to date

## References

1. Sutlive TG, Lopez HP, Schnitker DE, et al. Development of a clinical prediction rule for diagnosing hip osteoarthritis in individuals with unilateral hip pain. *J Orthop Sports Phys Ther*. 2008;38:542–550.

DIAGNOSTIC

## The American College of Rheumatology Criteria for the Classification of Osteoarthritis (OA) of the Knee[1]

**Diagnostic**

**Level: III**

Knee Osteoarthritis Present if:

**Three or More** Predictor Variables Present

**+LR 3.1**

**–LR 0.1**

Knee Osteoarthritis Present if:

**One or More** Predictor Variables **Plus** Osteophyte on Radiograph

**+LR 6.5**

**–LR 0.1**

### Predictor Variables

- Knee pain *plus* at least three of the six following items
  1. Age > 50
  2. Morning stiffness < 30 minutes
  3. Crepitus with active motion
  4. Bony tenderness
  5. Bony enlargement
  6. No palpable warmth

### Predictor Variables plus Radiography

- Knee pain *and* osteophytes on knee radiograph *plus* at least one of the following three clinical findings
  1. Age > 50
  2. Morning stiffness < 30 minutes
  3. Crepitus with active motion

### Clinical Bottom Line

There is a small shift in probability that patients with knee pain who meet three or more clinical predictor variables will have clinical OA. If osteophytes are seen on radiography and one or more predictor variables are present, there is a moderate shift in probability that the patient has clinical knee OA. There is a large shift in probability that patients who do not have at least three of the above clinical findings do not have knee OA. This rule has been validated and may be applied to practice within the confines of the study's parameters; however, further external, broad validation studies still need to be performed.

### Study Specifics

*Inclusion Criteria*

- Consecutive patients with knee OA and a comparison population were recruited
- Knee pain of any quality, duration, or periodicity

- Pain of articular origin
- Available current radiographs of the knee

*Exclusion Criteria*

- Referral from hip, spine, or pari-articular regions (anserine, prepatellar, infrapatellar bursa)
- Characteristics of secondary knee OA

*Patient Characteristics*

- N = 237 subjects
- 113 with idiopathic knee OA
  - 107 control patients
- Mean age in the OA group = 62 (+/− 1)
  - Female = 76%
  - Male = 24%
- Mean age in the control group = 47 (+/− 2)
  - Female = 69%
  - Male = 31%

*Definition of Positive (Reference Standard)*

- Clinical diagnosis of knee OA using all available findings from history, physical exam, labs, and diagnostic testing
  - Diagnosis was reviewed by three members of a subcommittee for verification of the diagnosis

*Validation*

- Internal validity of 50 patients with other rheumatic causes of knee pain demonstrated a Sn of 90% and a Sp of 71–84% using the "tree method" of analysis.[1]

## References

1. Altman R, Asch E, Bloch D, et al. Development of criteria for the classification and reporting of osteoarthritis: classification of osteoarthritis of the knee. *Arthritis Rheum.* 1986;29:1039–1049.

DIAGNOSTIC

# Diagnosis of Knee Effusion[1]

**Diagnostic**

**Level: IV**

Diagnostic for Knee Effusion if:

**Both** Predictor Variables Present

**+LR 3.6**

(95% CI 2.2–5.9)

## Predictor Variables

**1.** Self-noticed knee swelling
**2.** Positive Ballottement test

## Clinical Bottom Line

The presence of both predictor variables creates a small but sometimes clinically meaningful shift in probability that the patient possesses clinically significant effusion as diagnosed by Magnetic Resonance Imaging (MRI). A methodological quality analysis is suggested before implementing this CPR as a component of the best available evidence.

## Examination

- Ballottement test (**Figure 8.7**)
  - The patient was in the supine position. The clinician applied quick downward pressure through the patella using two or three fingers. The test was considered positive if the patella clicked or floated upward after trochlear impact.

**Figure 8.7**
Ballottement test.

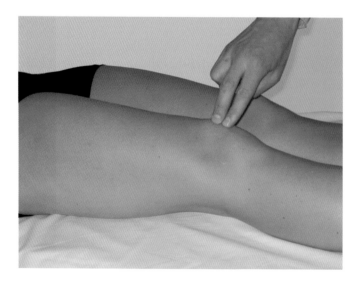

## Study Specifics

*Inclusion Criteria*

- Ages 18–65
- Traumatic knee complaints < 5 weeks before consultation

*Exclusion Criteria*

- Any contraindication to MRI (e.g., pregnancy, metal implants, pacemaker)

*Patient Characteristics*

- N = 134 subjects
- Mean age = 40.2 (+/− 12.2)
- Injury caused by sporting injury = 46%
- Percentage of patients defined as a clinically important effusion = 31%
  - 74% had an Anterior Cruciate Ligament (ACL) injury or meniscal tear
- Gender
  - Female = 45%
  - Male = 55%

*Definition of Positive (Reference Standard)*

- Effusion, as seen on the MRI, was defined as intra-articular fluid within the suprapatellar, medial, or lateral compartment. Rated as
  - Clinically important effusion (moderate or severe) was defined as fluid in all three compartments with or without bulging of the capsule and peri-capsular soft tissue as per the MRI

*Validation/Impact Analysis*

- None reported to date

## References

1. Kastelein M, Luijsterburg PA, Wagemakers HP, et al. Diagnostic value of history taking and physical examination to assess effusion of the knee in traumatic knee patients in general practice. *Arch Phys Med Rehabil.* 2009;90:82–86.

## DIAGNOSTIC

# Diagnosis of Medial Collateral Ligament (MCL) Tear for Patients with Knee Pain[1]

**Diagnostic**

**Level: IV**

Diagnostic for **Medial Collateral Ligament** Tear if:

**Both** Predictor Variables Present

**+LR 6.4**
(95% CI 2.7–15.2)

### Predictor Variables

1. History of external force to leg OR rotational trauma *and*
2. Pain *and* laxity with valgus stress test at 30°

### Clinical Bottom Line

The presence of both predictor variables creates a moderate shift in posttest probability that the patient possesses an MCL tear as diagnosed by an MRI. A methodological quality analysis is suggested before implementing this CPR as a component of the best available evidence.

### Examination

- History of external force to leg *or* rotational trauma:
  - Taken from subjective examination
- Valgus stress test at 30° (**Figure 8.8**)
  - The patient was in the supine position with his or her hip slightly abducted and the knee flexed to 30°. The clinician positioned one hand over the lateral aspect of the knee and grasped the ankle with the other hand. A valgus stress was applied. It was graded as positive if pain was elicited *and* laxity was noted compared to the opposite side.

**Figure 8.8**
Valgus stress test at 30°.

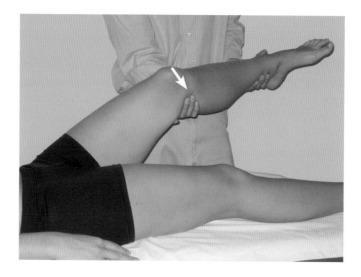

## Study Specifics

*Inclusion Criteria*

- Ages 18–65
- Traumatic knee complaints < 5 weeks before consultation

*Exclusion Criteria*

- Any MRI contraindications (e.g., pregnancy, metal implants, or pacemaker)

*Patient Characteristics*

- N = 134 subjects
- Mean age = 40.2 (+/− 12.2)
- Percentage of patients with MCL tear = 26%
  - 31% with clinically important effusion
- Injury caused by sporting injury = 46%
- Gender
  - Female = 45%
  - Male = 55%

*Definition of Positive (Reference Standard)*

- Medical collateral ligament tear as seen on a MRI

*Validation/Impact Analysis*

- None reported to date

## References

1. Kastelein M, Luijsterburg PA, Wagemakers HP, et al. Diagnostic value of history taking and physical examination to assess effusion of the knee in traumatic knee patients in general practice. *Arch Phys Med Rehabil*. 2009;90:82–86.

INTERVENTIONAL

# Lumbar Manipulation in Patellofemoral Pain Syndrome (PFPS)[1]

| | |
|---|---|
| **Interventional** | |
| **Level: IV** | |
| **Quality Score: 56%** | |

Lumbar Manipulation Indicated if:

**Three or More**
Predictor Variables
Present

**+LR 18.4**
(95% CI 3.6–105.3)

## Predictor Variables

1. Side-to-side hip internal rotation difference of > 14°
2. Ankle dorsiflexion with knee flexed > 16°
3. Navicular drop > 3 mm
4. No self-report stiffness with sitting > 20 minutes
5. Squatting reported as the most painful activity

## Clinical Bottom Line

The presence of three or more predictor variables creates a large and conclusive shift in probability that an individual will receive immediate benefit in either perceived global improvement and/or pain with functional testing after the lumbopelvic manipulation(s). The methodological quality of this study is below the suggested standard, so results should be taken with caution if this CPR is used clinically before validation.

## Examination

Figure 8.9
Hip internal rotation ROM with goniometer.

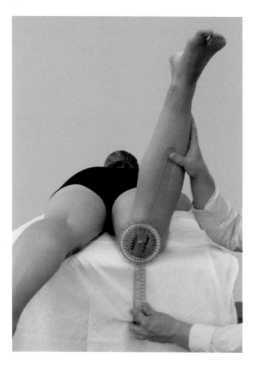

- Side-to-side hip internal rotation difference of > 14° (**Figure 8.9**)
  - The patient was in the prone position. The involved leg was placed in line with the body and the knee was flexed to 90°; the contralateral leg was slightly abducted. The axis of the goniometer was placed at the center of the knee, the stationary arm perpendicular to the ground, and the moving arm in line with the shaft of the tibia. The hip was passively internally rotated until the contralateral pelvis began to rise, and the measurement was taken.

- Ankle dorsiflexion > 16° (**Figure 8.10**)
  - The patient was in the prone position with the knee flexed. A goniometer was used with the stationary arm in line with the fibula, pointing at the fibular head. The moving arm was aligned with the fifth metatarsal and the axis just inferior to the lateral malleolus. The ankle was maximally dorsiflexed and the measurement was taken.

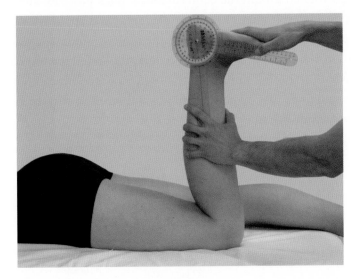

**Figure 8.10**
Ankle dorsiflexion
ROM with knee flexed
to 90°.

- Navicular drop > 3 mm (**Figure 8.11**)
  - The patient was in the standing position. A mark was made over the navicular tubercle, the patient was then placed in the subtalar neutral position, and a mark was made on an index card at the subsequent height. The patient was then asked to relax the calcaneal stance and a second recording was made on the card. The difference between the two marks was measured as the navicular drop.

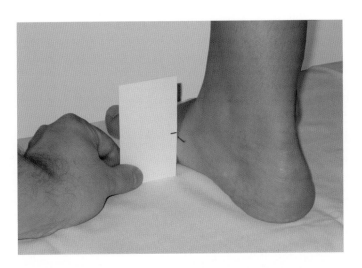

**Figure 8.11**
Navicular drop test.

## Intervention

Patients were treated for one session. Treatment included:

- Lumbopelvic manipulation (**Figure 8.12**)
  - The clinician stood opposite the side to be manipulated. The patient was passively side bent away from the clinician. The patient's trunk was then passively rotated toward the clinician and a quick posterior and inferior thrust through the anterior superior iliac spine was applied.
  - Manipulation was first performed on the most symptomatic side. If a cavitation was noted during the procedure, the technique was complete. If a cavitation was not noted, the technique was performed a second time on the same side. If a cavitation still was not heard or felt, the manipulation was administered to the opposite side.

**Figure 8.12**
Lumbopelvic manipulation.

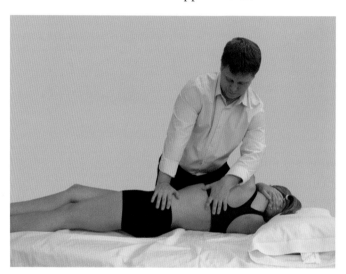

## Study Specifics

*Inclusion Criteria*

- Military health care beneficiaries
- Ages 18–50
- Clinical diagnosis of PFPS
  - Anterior knee pain provoked with two of the following: squatting, stair ascent, stair descent, prolonged sitting, kneeling, or isometric quadriceps contraction

## Exclusion Criteria

- Pregnancy
- Signs of nerve root compression
- Tenderness over the tibiofemoral joint lines or patellar tendon
- Positive special tests for knee ligament of meniscal injuries
- Prior surgery to the spine or symptomatic knee
- Osteoporosis
- Compression fracture
- History of systemic, connective tissue, or neurological disease
- Currently receiving other treatments for the knee

## Patient Characteristics

- N = 49 subjects
- Mean age = 24.5 (+/– 6.8)
- Percentage of patients defined as a treatment success = 45%
- Mean duration of symptoms (weeks) = 94.9 (+/– 193.4)
- Gender
  - Female = 47%
  - Male = 53%

## Definition of Success

- ≥ 50% improvement on the composite of score with stair ascent, descent, and squatting *or*
- ≥ + 4 (moderately better) on the GROC score

## Validation/Impact Analysis

- None reported to date

## References

1. Iverson CA, Sutlive TG, Crowell MS, et al. Lumbopelvic manipulation for the treatment of patients with patellofemoral pain syndrome: development of a clinical prediction rule. *J Orthop Sports Phys Ther.* 2008;38:297–312.

## INTERVENTIONAL

# Patellar Taping for Patellofemoral Pain Syndrome (PFPS)[1]

**Interventional**

**Level: IV**

**Quality Score: 67%**

Patellar Taping
Indicated if:

**One or More** Predictor
Variables Present

**+LR 4.4**
(95% CI 1.3–12.3)

### Predictor Variables

**1.** Tibial varum > 5°
**2.** Positive patellar tilt test

### Clinical Bottom Line

The presence of either of the two identified predictor variables creates a small but sometimes clinically important shift in probability that an individual will receive immediate benefit in either perceived global improvement and/or a ≥ 50% reduction in pain after medial patellar taping. The methodological quality of the derivation study was acceptable; therefore, it is appropriate to use this CPR as a component of the best available evidence.

### Examination

- Tibial varum > 5° (**Figure 8.13**)
  - A line was drawn on the patient bisecting the affected Achilles' tendon. The patient was in the standing position on a step in relaxed stance. A goniometer was used to measure the angle between the horizontal surface of the stool and the line bisecting the Achilles tendon.

**Figure 8.13**
Measurement of tibial varum.

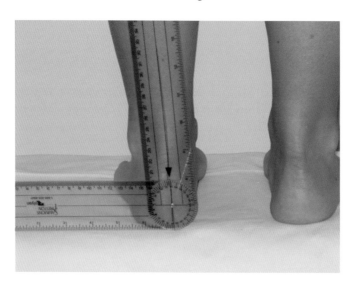

- Positive patellar tilt test (Figure 8.14)
  - The patient was in the supine position with muscles in the leg relaxed. The clinician passively glided the patella laterally and attempted to lift the lateral border of the patella anteriorly. The variable was considered positive if the lateral border could be lifted above the horizontal plane.

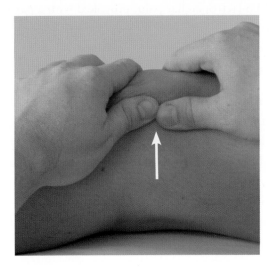

**Figure 8.14**
Patellar tilt test.

## Intervention

Patients were treated for one session. Treatment included:

- Patellar tapping (Figure 8.15)
  - A single piece of leukotape was placed over the lateral aspect of the patella and pulled from lateral to medial.

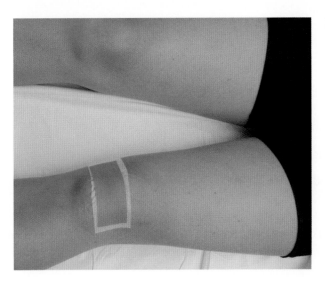

**Figure 8.15**
Patellar taping.

## Study Specifics

*Inclusion Criteria*

- Military health care beneficiaries
- Ages 18–50
- Clinical diagnosis of PFPS (retropatellar pain, provoked with a partial squat or stair ascent/descent)
- Fluent in English

*Exclusion Criteria*

- Abnormal neurological status
- Recent history of knee trauma
- Ligamentous laxity of the painful knee
- Tenderness of the joint lines or patellar tendon
- Prior knee surgery on symptomatic knee
- Systemic disease, neurologic disease, or connective tissue disease
- Additional lower extremity conditions (e.g., stress fractures, shin splints)
- Already receiving treatment for knee pain

*Patient Characteristics*

- N = 50 subjects
- Mean age = 22.8 (+/– 4.2)
- Percentage of subjects defined as a successful outcome = 52%
- Mean duration of symptoms (days) = 75.4 (+/– 123.8)
- Gender
  - Female = 46%
  - Male = 54%

*Definition of Success*

- ≥ 50% improvement on the composite NPRS of the functional tests (stepping up onto a 20-cm step, stepping down from a 20-cm step, and squatting) *or*
- ≥ + 4 (moderately better) on the GROC score

*Validation/Impact Analysis*

- None reported to date

## References

1. Lesher JD, Sutlive TG, Miller GA, Chine NJ, Garber MB, Wainner RS. Development of a clinical prediction rule for classifying patients with patellofemoral pain syndrome who respond to patellar taping. *J Orthop Sports Phys Ther.* 2006;36:854–866.

## INTERVENTIONAL

# Orthotics in Patients with Patellofemoral Pain Syndrome (PFPS)[1]

## Predictor Variables

1. Age > 25
2. Height < 165 cm
3. Worst pain < 53.25 mm on 100 mm VAS
4. Midfoot width difference > 10.96 mm
   a. Measured with a digital caliper in weight bearing and nonweightbearing position
   b. Measurement was taken at 50% of the foot length

## Clinical Bottom Line

Patients who possess three or more of the predictor variables have a moderate shift in probability that they will experience "marked improvement" in their condition after 12 weeks of orthotic use. The methodological quality of this study is below the suggested standard, so results should be taken with caution if this CPR is used clinically before validation.

## Intervention

Patients were treated for six sessions over 6 weeks. Treatment included:
- Foot orthoses
  - Prefabricated ethylene-vinyl acetate (EVA) foot orthoses with 6° varus wedge and arch support inbuilt
  - PT selected EVA densities
  - PT selected modifications including heat molding, and wedge and heel raise additions

## Study Specifics

### Inclusion Criteria

- Ages 18–40
- Anterior or retropatellar knee pain of nontraumatic origin greater than 6-weeks duration
- Provoked by at least two predefined activities
  - Prolonged sitting
  - Squatting
  - Jogging or running

**Interventional**

**Level: IV**

**Quality Score: 50%**

Orthotics Indicated if:

**Three or More** Predictor Variables Present

**+LR 8.8** (95% CI 1.2–66.9)

- Hopping
- Jumping
- Stair walking
- Pain on palpation of the patellar facets or with step down from a 25-cm step or double-leg squat
- Pain over the previous week of at least 30 mm on a 100 mm VAS

*Exclusion Criteria*

- Concomitant injury of pathology of other knee structures
- Previous knee surgery
- Patellofemoral instability
  - History of subluxation or dislocation
  - Positive apprehension test
- Knee joint effusion
- Osgood–Schlatter's disease
- Sinding–Larsen–Johanssen disease
- Any foot condition that precluded use of foot orthoses
- Hip or lumbar spine pain (local or referred)
- Physiotherapy within previous year
- Prior foot orthoses treatment
- Use of anti-inflammatories or corticosteroids

*Patient Characteristics*

- N = 42 subjects
- Mean age = 27.9 (+/– 5.5)
- Percentage of subjects defined as success = 40%
- Gender
  - Female = 57%
  - Male = 43%

*Definition of Positive*

- Perceived "marked improvement" on a 5-point Likert scale consisting of marked improvement, moderate improvement, same, moderate worsening, and marked worsening

*Validation/Impact Analysis*

- None reported to date

## References

1. Vicenzino B, Collins N, Cleland J, McPoil T. A clinical prediction rule for identifying patients with patellofemoral pain who are likely to benefit from foot orthoses: a preliminary determination. *Br J Sports Med.* 2008;Epub ahead of print.

## INTERVENTIONAL

# Prefabricated Orthotics and Modified Activity for Individuals with Patellofemoral Pain Syndrome (PFPS)[1]

## Predictor Variables

1. Forefoot valgus ≥ 2°
2. Great toe extension ≤ 78°
3. Navicular drop ≤ 3 mm

## Clinical Bottom Line

The presence of one or more predictor variables creates a small but sometimes clinically important shift in probability that the patient will benefit (decreased pain by ≥ 50%) from orthotics and activity modification at 3 weeks. The methodological quality of the derivation study was acceptable; therefore, it is appropriate to use this CPR as a component of the best available evidence.

## Examination

- Forefoot valgus ≥ 2° (**Figure 8.16**)
  - Measured with the patient in the prone position, foot subtalar neutral position.

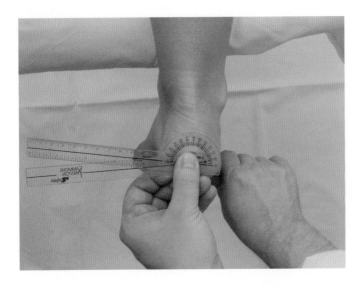

**Figure 8.16**
Measurement of forefoot valgus in prone position.

**Interventional**

**Level: IV**

**Quality Score: 61%**

Orthotics indicated if:

**One or More** Predictor Variables Present

**Forefoot Valgus:**
**+LR 4.0**
(95% CI 0.7–21.9)

**Great Toe Extension:**
**+LR 4.0** (95% CI 0.7–21.9)

**Navicular Drop:**
**+LR 2.3**
(95% CI 1.3–4.3)

- Great toe extension ≤ 78° (**Figure 8.17**)
  - The patient was in the long sitting position. The proximal arm of the goniometer was placed along the first metatarsal, the axis over the metatarsophalangeal (MTP) joint, and the distal arm along the toe. The measurement was passive.

**Figure 8.17**
Measurement of great toe extension.

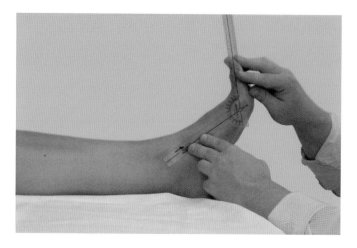

- Navicular drop ≤ 3 mm (**Figure 8.18**)
  - The patient was in the standing-on-a-step position. A mark was made over the navicular tubercle. The patient was then placed in the subtalar neutral position and a mark was made on an index card at the subsequent height. The patient was then asked to relax the calcaneal stance and a second recording was made on the card. The difference between the two marks was measured as the navicular drop.

**Figure 8.18**
Navicular drop test.

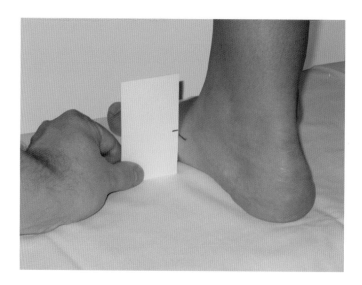

## Intervention

Patients were treated for two sessions over 21 days. Treatment included:

- Prefabricated orthotics with a full arch support and a firm heel cushion were issued to be worn at all times.
- Instructions including limiting squatting, kneeling, and deep-knee bends as well as walking distance, running for the first 7 days, and no lower-body-resistance exercise.

## Study Specifics

### Inclusion Criteria

- Symptoms of PFPS (retropatellar pain that increases with weight-bearing activities such as running, squatting, or stairs)
- Fluent in English

### Exclusion Criteria

- Recent trauma to the knee
- Ligamentous laxity of the knee
- History of surgery to the affected knee
- Systemic or neurological disease
- Other lower extremity conditions (shin splints, stress fractures)
- Already receiving treatment for the knee

### Patient Characteristics

- N = 45 subjects, 78 knees
- Mean age = 28.1 (+/− 6.2)
- Percentage of subjects defined as a treatment success = 60%
- Mean duration of symptoms (weeks) = 173.6 (+/− 190.7)
- Gender
  - Female = 24%
  - Male = 76%

### Definition of Success

- ≥ 50% improvement on the VAS

### Validation/Impact Analysis

- None reported to date

## References

1. Sutlive TG, Mitchell SD, Maxfield SN, et al. Identification of individuals with patellofemoral pain whose symptoms improved after a combined program of foot orthosis use and modified activity: a preliminary investigation. *Phys Ther*. 2004;84:49–61.

INTERVENTIONAL

# Hip Mobilization in Knee Osteoarthritis (OA)[1]

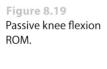

**Interventional**

**Level: IV**

**Quality Score: 56%**

Hip Mobilization
Indicated if:

**Two or More** Predictor
Variables Present

**+LR 12.9**
(95% CI 0.8–205.6)

## Predictor Variables

**1.** Ipsilateral hip or groin pain or paresthesias
**2.** Ipsilateral anterior thigh pain
**3.** Ipsilateral passive knee flexion < 122°
**4.** Ipsilateral passive hip medial rotation < 17°
**5.** Pain with ipsilateral hip distraction

## Clinical Bottom Line

The presence of two or more predictor variables creates a large and conclusive shift in probability that an individual with knee OA will receive short-term (48-hour) benefits in either perceived global improvement and/or pain with functional tests after hip mobilizations with the implementation of hip mobilizations and exercise. The methodological quality of this study is below the suggested standard, so results should be taken with caution if this CPR is used clinically before validation.

## Examination

- Ipsilateral passive knee flexion < 122° (**Figure 8.19**)
    - Measured in the supine position with a goniometer with the axis at the greater trochanter, stationary arm toward the midaxillary line, and moving arm in line with the shaft of the femur pointed at the lateral epicondyle.

**Figure 8.19**
Passive knee flexion
ROM.

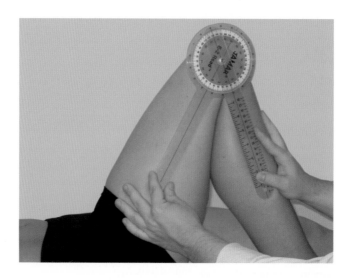

- Ipsilateral passive hip medial rotation < 17° (**Figure 8.20**)
  - Measured in the prone position with the knee flexed and the opposite leg slightly abducted. The lower leg was placed vertical, and the inclinometer was placed just below the lateral malleoli and adjusted to zero. The lower leg was rotated into internal rotation until the opposite hip began to rise off of the table.

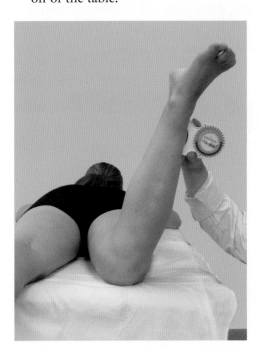

**Figure 8.20**
Hip internal rotation ROM with inclinometer.

**Figure 8.21**
Hip distraction test.

- Pain with ipsilateral hip distraction (**Figure 8.21**)
  - The patient was in the supine position with the involved lower extremity held between the therapist's axilla. One hand was held above the knee and the other was held on the lower leg. The leg was positioned in 30° of flexion, abduction, and external rotation. The clinician leaned backwards and assessed the patient's response.

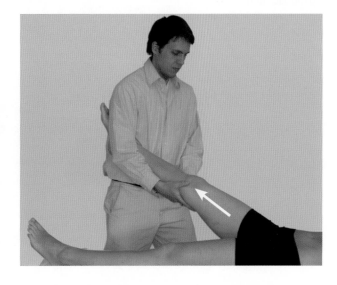

## Intervention

Patients were treated for one session. Treatment included:

- Hip mobilizations
  - A caudal glide with a belt (Figure 8.22), as well as an A-P glide were applied in the supine position (Figure 8.23). A P-A glide (Figure 8.24) as well as a P-A glide in flexion, abduction, and external rotation (FABER) (Figure 8.25) were applied in the prone position. Mobilizations were grade IV and three sets of 30 seconds were applied.

**Figure 8.22**
Caudal glide mobilization with belt.

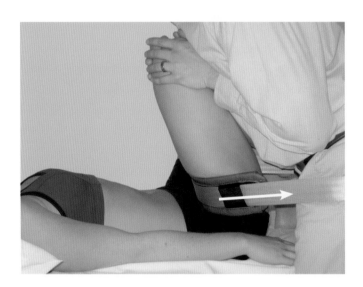

**Figure 8.23**
Anterior to posterior hip mobilization.

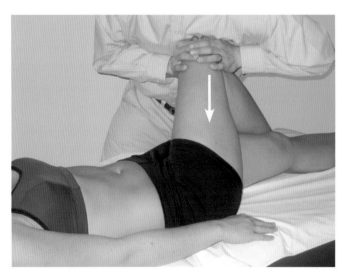

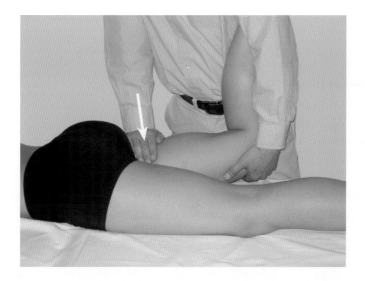

**Figure 8.24**
Posterior to anterior
hip mobilization.

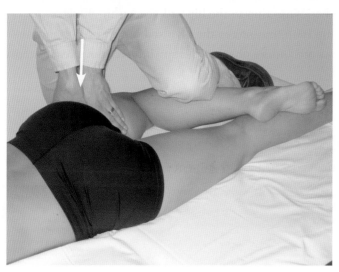

**Figure 8.25**
Posterior to anterior
hip mobilization in
FABER position.

- Home exercise
  - Instructed in the supine hip flexion position, within the patient's comfortable range of motion, for two repetitions of 30 seconds, twice per day.

## Study Specifics

*Inclusion Criteria*

- Ages 50–80
- Eligible for military health care
- Sufficient English skills to comprehend all explanations
- Primary complaint of knee pain

- ≥ 3 of the following (Altman Criteria)[2]
  - > 50 years old
  - Knee crepitus
  - Palpable bony enlargement
  - Bony tenderness to palpation
  - < 30 minutes of morning stiffness
  - No palpable warmth of the synovium

*Exclusion Criteria*

- Primary complaint of low back pain
- Secondary complaint of low back pain with pain radiating below the knee
- Osteoporosis
- History of cancer
- History of hip or knee arthroplasty
- Cortisone or synthetic injection to the hip or knee within 30 days
- History of prior hip mobilizations to the involved limb within 6 months
- Current conditions precluding physical therapy interventions (e.g., deep-vein thrombosis)

*Patient Characteristics*

- N = 60 subjects
- Mean age = 65.8 (+/− 7.2)
- Percentage of patients defined as a treatment success = 68%
- Gender
  - Female = 45%
  - Male = 55%

*Definition of Success*

- ≥ 30% improvement on the composite Numerical Pain Rating Scale (squat test and sit to stand from a chair) *or*
- ≥ + 3 on the GROC score

*Validation/Impact Analysis*

- None reported to date

## References

1. Currier LL, Froehlich PJ, Carow SD, et al. Development of a clinical prediction rule to identify patients with knee pain and clinical evidence of knee osteoarthritis who demonstrate a favorable short-term response to hip mobilization. *Phys Ther*. 2007;87:1106–1119.
2. Altman R, Asch E, Bloch D, et al. For the diagnostic and therapeutic criteria committee of the American Rheumatism Association. Development of criteria for the classification and reporting of osteoarthritis: classification of osteoarthritis of the knee. *Arthritis Rheum*. 1986;29:1039–1049.

INTERVENTIONAL

# Manual Therapy and Exercise After Inversion Ankle Sprain[1]

## Predictor Variables

1. Symptoms worse with standing
2. Symptoms worse in the evening
3. Navicular drop ≥ 5.0 mm
4. Distal tibiofibular joint hypomobility

## Clinical Bottom Line

The presence of three predictor variables creates a moderate shift in probability that the individual post-inversion ankle sprain will experience moderate perceived global improvement from manual therapy and exercise within two treatment sessions (4–8 days). The methodological quality of the derivation study was acceptable; therefore, it is appropriate to use this CPR as a component of the best available evidence.

**Interventional**

**Level: IV**

**Quality Score: 83%**

Manual Therapy and Exercise Indicated if:

**Three or More** Predictor Variables Present

**+LR 5.9** (95% CI 1.1–41.6)

## Examination

- Navicular drop ≥ 5.0 mm (**Figure 8.26**)
  - The patient was in the standing position. A mark was made over the navicular tubercle and the patient was placed in the subtalar neutral position. The navicular height was then recorded on an index card. The patient then relaxed the calacaneal stance and a second recording was made on the card. The difference between the two marks was measured, indicating the navicular drop.

**Figure 8.26**
Navicular drop test.

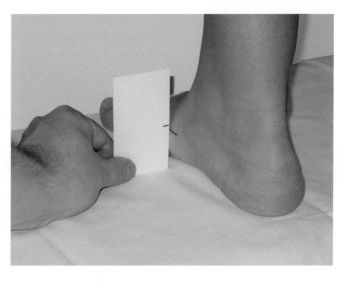

- Distal tibiofibular joint hypomobility (**Figure 8.27**)
  - The patient was in the supine position. The clinician stabilized the distal tibia with one hand while gliding the distal fibula via pressure over the medial malleolus.

**Figure 8.27**
Distal tibiofibular joint mobility assessment.

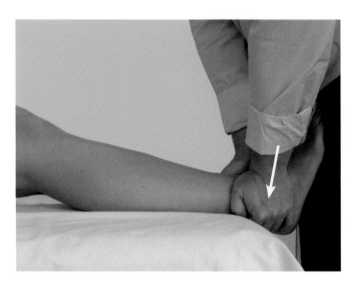

---

## Intervention

Patients were treated for one to two sessions over 4–8 days. Treatment included:

- Manual treatment
  - Rear foot distraction thrust manipulation (**Figure 8.28**)
    - The patient was in the supine position. The clinician placed his or her hands around the dorsum of the foot. The foot was dorsiflexed and everted until the restrictive barrier was felt. The thrust manipulation was then applied in the caudal direction.
  - Proximal tibiofibular posteroanterior thrust manipulation (**Figure 8.29**)
    - The patient was in the hook-lying position. The clinician placed his or her second metacarpalphalangeal joint (MCP) in the popliteal space and pulled laterally until his or her MCP was behind the posterior fibula. The foot and ankle were grasped, the knee was flexed, and the distal leg was externally rotated until the restrictive barrier was felt behind the fibula. A posterior-directed thrust manipulation was applied into knee flexion.

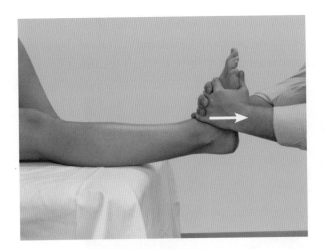

**Figure 8.28**
Rear-foot distraction manipulation.

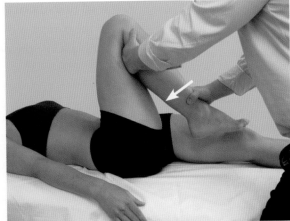

**Figure 8.29**
Proximal tibiofibular posteroanterior manipulation.

- Anterior to posterior (A-P) talocrural non-thrust manipulation (**Figure 8.30**)
  - The patient was in the supine position. The patient's foot was on the clinician's anterior thigh to adjust the dorsiflexion range of motion. One hand stabilized the distal tibiofibular joint while the other hand imparted a posterior force through the anterior talus.
- Lateral glide of the rear foot (talocrural and subtalar joint) (**Figure 8.31**)
  - The patient was in the side-lying position. The clinician stabilized the distal tibiofibular joint with one hand while the other imparted a lateral force through the talus. The technique was then repeated while stabilizing the talus and mobilizing the calcaneus.

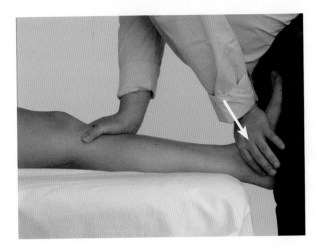

**Figure 8.30**
Anterior to posterior talocrural mobilization.

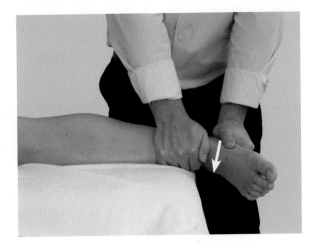

**Figure 8.31**
Side-lying lateral subtalar mobilization.

■ Distal tibiofibular A-P mobilization (**Figure 8.32**)
  ● The patient was in the supine position. One hand stabilized the distal tibia while the other imparted an A-P force through the distal fibula.

**Figure 8.32**
Distal tibiofibular anterior to posterior mobilization.

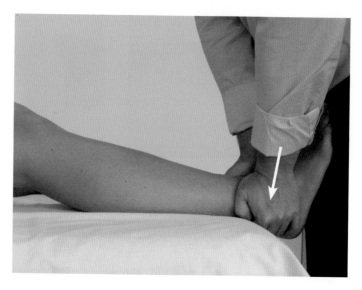

● Exercise
  ■ Achilles' tendon stretch (weight bearing and non-weight bearing)
    ● Non-weight-bearing stretching was performed in the long-sitting position by utilizing a towel to impart a dorsiflexion motion with the knee straight (**Figure 8.33**).

**Figure 8.33**
Dorsiflexion stretch in the long-sitting position.

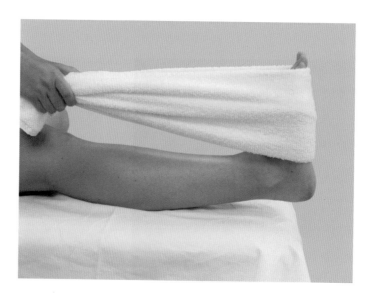

- Weight-bearing stretching was performed in the standing position with the knee extended. The Achilles tendon to be stretched was placed behind the other foot and a forward lunge position was performed (**Figure 8.34**).
- Alphabet exercises
  - The patient moved his or her foot and ankle to draw each letter of the alphabet.
- Ankle self-eversion mobilization (**Figure 8.35**)
  - The patient was sitting with the foot to be mobilized crossed over the opposite leg at the thigh. The patient used one hand to stabilize the distal tibiofibular joint while the other hand applied a medial–to–lateral force through the calcaneus.
- Dorsiflexion self-mobilization
  - Performed similar to the Achilles stretch except the knee was flexed and a self-mobilization was performed (**Figure 8.36**).

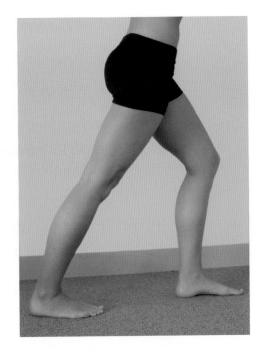

**Figure 8.34**
(Above) Weight-bearing dorsiflexion stretch—knee extended.

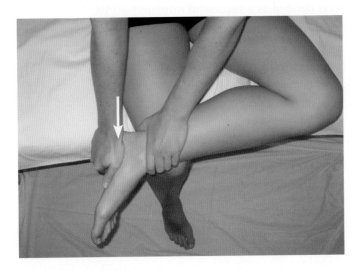

**Figure 8.35**
Self-lateral calcaneal glide in the sitting position.

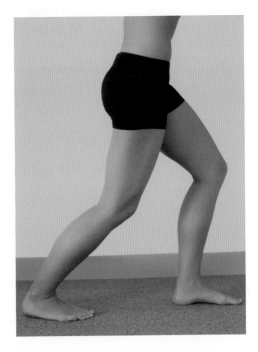

**Figure 8.36**
Dorsiflexion self-mobilization—knee flexed.

## Study Specifics

### Inclusion Criteria

- Ages 18–60
- Primary report of ankle pain
- Grade I or II inversion ankle sprain over the past year
- NPRS indicating worst pain over the past week > 3/10
- Negative Ottawa Ankle Rules (no need for radiographs)

### Exclusion Criteria

- Red flags including tumor, rheumatoid arthritis, osteoporosis, prolonged steroid use, severe vascular disease, and so on
- Prior surgery to the distal tibia, fibula, ankle joint, or rear-foot region
- Grade III ankle sprains
- Fracture
- Any other absolute contraindications to manual therapy

### Patient Characteristics

- N = 85 subjects
- Mean age = 32 (+/− 14.1)
- Percentage of subjects defined as a successful outcome = 75%
- Mean duration of symptoms (days) = 22.3 (+/− 43.9)
  - Median: 11 days
- Gender
  - Female = 49%
  - Male = 51%

### Definition of Success

- ≥ +5 (quite a bit better) on the GROC score

### Validation/Impact Analysis

- None reported to date

## References

1. Whitman JM, Cleland JA, Mintken P, et al. Predicting short-term response to thrust and non-thrust manipulation and exercise in patients post inversion ankle sprain. *J Orthop Sports Phys Ther*. 2009;39:188–200.

# CHAPTER 9

# CASE STUDIES

We have included the following case studies to provide the reader with examples of how clinical prediction rules may be used in the broader context of clinical decision making. The information contained in these case studies is intended to provide general guidelines for the implementation of CPRs at various levels of development. You can also refer to the CPR decision-making flow chart we have provided in Appendix E for a visual representation of the thought process.

These case studies are not intended to encompass the full breadth of the literature but rather to indicate instances where CPRs can facilitate evidence-based diagnosis, treatment, or prognosis. They are reminders that CPRs are intended to be one of the many aspects of clinical decision making and should not be used as the ultimate decision tool.

## CASE STUDY

# Cervicothoracic Spine

### Historical Exam

A 52-year-old, right-handed, female high school teacher presenting to physical therapy 3 weeks after insidious onset of left-sided neck pain as well as shoulder and arm pain down to the first three digits.

**Past medical history (PMH):** Noncontributory

**Aggravating factors:** Cervical extension, left rotation, and left side bending

**Relieving factors:** Supine position, ibuprofen

| Self-Report Outcome Measures | |
|---|---|
| Neck Disability Index (NDI) | 34% |
| Fear Avoidance Belief Questionnaire Work Subscale (FABQ-W) | 14 |
| Fear Avoidance Belief Questionnaire Physical Activity Subscale (FABQ-PA) | 8 |
| Patient Specific Functional Scale (PSFS) | 12 |

### Physical Exam

**Negative tests:** Sharp–Purser Test, Hoffman's Sign, Vertebrobasilar artery insufficiency test, dermatomal, myotomal, and reflex testing were within normal limits

**Positive tests:** Spurling's A Test, ULTT A, Cervical Distraction Test, Shoulder Abduction Sign

**Posture:** Slight forward head posture with rounded shoulders and decreased upper-thoracic kyphosis

| Cervical Active Range of Motion (Inclinometer) | |
|---|---|
| Extension | 25° with provocation of arm pain |
| Flexion | 55° symptoms status quo |
| Right side bending | 40° symptoms status quo |
| Left side bending | 30° with provocation of left-sided neck and shoulder pain |

| Cervical Active Range of Motion (Goniometer) | |
|---|---|
| Right cervical rotation | 80° symptoms status quo |
| Left cervical rotation | 50° with provocation of arm pain |

**Craniocervical flexion test:** 26mm Hg held for 8 seconds per pressure biofeedback unit

**Passive intervertebral motion:** Left-sided mid- and lower-cervical hypomobility with reproduction of the patient's comparable symptoms during lower-cervical assessment.

## Clinical Decision Making

### Diagnosis/Classification

Wainner et al.[1] derived a diagnostic CPR for the clinical diagnosis of cervical radiculopathy. In the current case, the patient meets all four predictor criteria resulting in a large and conclusive shift in the posttest probability of the diagnosis of cervical radiculopathy.[1]

| Predictor Variables[1] | Variable Present |
|---|---|
| Ipsilateral cervical rotation < 60° | Yes |
| Positive ULTT A | Yes |
| Positive Spurling's A test | Yes |
| Positive cervical distraction test | Yes |

## Prognosis

The patient's likely prognosis can be predicted with the use of a CPR derived by Cleland et al.[2] The patient meets three of the four predictor variables thus producing a moderate shift in probability that a clinically meaningful change in outcomes will be achieved within 4 weeks.[2] Based upon the findings of Cleland et al,[2] the patient's prognosis can be further improved through the addition of multimodal treatment including traction, manual therapy, and deep-neck flexor strengthening. Lastly, additional positive prognostic indicators include the patient's young age and lack of comorbidities.

| Predictor Variables[2] | Variable Present |
|---|---|
| Age < 54 | Yes |
| Dominant arm is not affected | Yes |
| Looking down does not worsen symptoms | Yes |
| Received multimodal treatment | Will receive |

## Interventions

Cervical traction: This patient has been classified into the centralization subgroup due to the reproduction of her upper extremity symptoms.[3,4] She meets four of the five criteria identified by Raney et al,[5] indicating a large and conclusive shift in probability that she will benefit from mechanical traction.

| Predictor Variables[5] | Variable Present |
|---|---|
| Peripheralization with lower-cervical mobilizations | Yes |
| Positive shoulder abduction test | Yes |
| Age ≥ 55 | No |
| Positive ULTT A (median nerve bias) | Yes |
| Relief of symptoms with manual distraction | Yes |

Thoracic manipulation: This patient may be concurrently classified into the hypomobility subgroup as four out of six variables were met, indicating a large shift in probability that the patient will benefit from thoracic manipulation.[6]

| Predictor Variables[6] | Variable Present |
|---|---|
| Symptoms < 30 days | Yes |
| No symptoms distal to the shoulder | No |
| Looking up does not aggravate symptoms | No |
| FABQ-PA < 12 | Yes |
| Diminished upper-thoracic spine kyphosis | Yes |
| Cervical extension ROM < 30° | Yes |

**Deep-neck flexor strengthening:** Pressure biofeedback testing has indicated a lack of deep-neck flexor endurance. Currently, a prediction rule does not exist to identify individuals who may benefit from deep-neck flexor training; however, it has been identified as an important component in the treatment of individuals with cervical radiculopathy.[4,7]

## Discussion

All of the CPRs included in the clinical decision making for this case are Level IV in development, thus requiring careful consideration of multiple factors prior to incorporating them into the management of this patient. First, the methodological quality of each rule should be assessed to confirm it has limited bias. Second, the characteristics of the study sample should be analyzed to determine their resemblance to the patient in question. Finally, the study's statistical parameters (i.e., likelihood ratios) should be considered to determine the magnitude and direction of probability shift and whether this shift surpasses the treatment threshold.

The four CPRs used to help guide clinical decision making in this case possess quality scores of greater than 60%, indicating "high" or acceptable levels of quality.[8,9] The subject's age and gender are similar to the populations studied within the CPRs in question. Additionally, the patient meets the inclusion criteria and would not be excluded from any of the CPRs. The duration of this episode of neck pain, 3 weeks, suggests she may be slightly more acute than the typical subject in the derivation studies for these CPRs; however, related research indicates greater improvements with manual therapy in individuals who are acute, thus this would not be a reason to abandon the use of these CPRs in the clinical decision making.[6]

The location and behavior of symptoms are characteristic of cervical radiculopathy and suggest an initial treatment-based classification into the centralization subgroup.[3] The CPR for cervical radiculopathy provides further support for this decision.[1] The determination of a favorable prognosis for this patient was established through the use of the CPR by Cleland et al.[6] The individual in this case met three of the four variables, identifying a moderate shift in probability that she will significantly improve within 4 weeks. This CPR also begins to direct treatment as it indicates the improved likelihood of success with the implementation of a multimodal treatment approach.

Treatment based on the patient's status on two CPRs indicates the potential benefit of thoracic manipulation and cervical traction.[5,6] The patient meets four variables on both CPRs, creating large and conclusive shifts in probability that she will benefit from these interventions. Despite these findings, the clinician must remember that the confidence intervals in both instances were wide with the lower end indicating a small shift in probability. For this reason it is important that the decision to incorporate these interventions be confirmed from further research. In this case, recent evidence has demonstrated the benefit of a multimodal treatment approach for patients with cervical radiculopathy.[4,7]

By incorporating clinical prediction rules in the management of this patient, the diagnosis (cervical radiculopathy), prognosis (positive), and intervention plan (multimodal treatment) were efficiently and effectively achieved. These tools allow the clinician to refine his or her clinical decision making and improve his or her level of confidence in these decisions. The methodological quality was considered as were the statistical parameters of the rules. Interventions with strong evidence were used in conjunction with the CPR findings to formulate a comprehensive plan of care for the patient. Despite the high quality of the current Level IV CPRs and the strength of the existing literature further confirming the CPR findings, the management of this patient will include frequent reexamination of impairments and functional level outcomes to determine the validity of the diagnosis, the effectiveness of the intervention, and the accuracy of the prognosis.

## References

1. Wainner RS, Fritz JM, Irrgang JJ, Boninger ML, Delitto A, Allison S. Reliability and diagnostic accuracy of the clinical examination and patient self-report measures for cervical radiculpathy. *Spine.* 2003;28:52–62.

2. Cleland JA, Fritz JM, Whitman JM, Heath R. Predictors of short-term outcome in people with a clinical diagnosis of cervical radiculopathy. *Phys Ther.* 2007;87:1619–1632.

3. Childs JD, Fritz JM, Piva SR, Whitman JM. Proposal of a classification system for patients with neck pain. *J Orthop Sports Phys Ther.* 2004;34:686–696.

4. Childs JD, Cleland JA, Elliott JM, et al. Neck pain: clinical practice guidelines linked to the international classification of functioning, disability, and health from the orthopedic section of the American Physical Therapy Association. *J Orthop Sports Phys Ther.* 2008;38:A1–A34.

5. Raney NH, Petersen EJ, Smith TA, et al. Development of a clinical prediction rule to identify patients with neck pain likely to benefit from cervical traction and exercise. *Eur Spine J.* 2009;18:382–391.

6. Cleland JA, Childs JD, Fritz JM, Whitman JM, Eberhart SL. Development of a clinical prediction rule for guiding treatment of a subgroup of patients with neck pain: use of thoracic spine manipulation, exercise, and patient education. *Phys Ther.* 2007;878:9–23.

7. Cleland JA, Whitman JM, Fritz JM, Palmer JA. Manual physical therapy, cervical traction, and strengthening exercises in patients with cervical radiculopathy: a case series. *J Orthop Sports Phys Ther.* 2005;35:802–811.

8. Beneciuk JM, Bishop MD, George SZ. Clinical prediction rules for physical therapy interventions: a systematic review. *Phys Ther.* 2009;89:114–124.

9. Kuijpers T, van der Windt DAWM, van der Heijden GJMG, Bouter LM. Systematic review of prognostic cohort studies on shoulder disorders. *Pain.* 2004;109:420–431.

## CASE STUDY

# Knee

### Historical Exam

A 43-year-old recreational runner with a 6-week history of worsening left anterior knee pain. She reports an insidious onset of retropatellar and infrapatellar pain. It is now limiting her ability to continue running and comfortably descend stairs.

**Aggravating factors:** Squatting, sitting with bent knee greater than 30 minutes, running greater than 10 minutes, descending stairs

**Relieving factors:** Rest, ice, ibuprofen, frequent position changes

**PMH:** Noncontributory

| Self-Report Outcome Measures | |
| --- | --- |
| Lower Extremity Functional Scale (LEFS) | 52/80 |
| Numeric Pain Rating Scale (NPRS): Current | 2/10 left anterior knee |
| Numeric Pain Rating Scale (NPRS): Worst in past 24 hours | 5/10 left anterior knee |
| Numeric Pain Rating Scale (NPRS): Best in past 24 hours | 0/10 |

### Physical Exam

**Observation:** 5'2" (157 cm) otherwise healthy and athletic female; mild bilateral infrapatellar swelling

**Posture (standing):** Bilateral genu valgus and genu recurvatum; bilateral patella alta; bilateral calcaneal valgus

**Gait:** Bilateral and symmetrical excessive pronation with late supination (left greater than right)

**Palpation:** Tenderness to palpation at the inferior patellar pole of the left patella; no other tenderness to palpation noted

**Range of motion (ROM):** Bilateral knee ROM within normal limits (WNL)

| Regional ROM Measurements | Right | Left |
|---|---|---|
| Hip Internal Rotation PROM[1] | 40° | 24° |
| Ankle Dorsiflexion AROM[1] | 20° | 20° |
| Great Toe Extension PROM[2] | 80° | 80° |
| Navicular Drop[1] | 6 mm | 8 mm |
| Forefoot Valgus[2] | 0° | 0° |
| Tibial Varum[3] | 7° | 8° |

**Manual muscle test:** 4/5 in the left hip external rotators and abductors; otherwise 5/5 and painfree throughout the bilateral LEs

| Anthropometric Measurements | Right | Left |
|---|---|---|
| Mid-foot width[4] Weight bearing | 74 mm | 76 mm |
| Mid-foot width[4] Non-weight bearing | 63 mm | 64 mm |

| Special Tests | Right | Left |
|---|---|---|
| Patellar tilt test[3] | Negative | Positive |
| Eccentric step down test[5] | WNL | Hip adduction and internal rotation |
| VMO coordination test[5] | Negative | Positive |
| Patellar apprehension test[5] | Negative | Positive |

# Clinical Decision Making

## Diagnosis

**Appropriateness for PT:** There are no indications of trauma from the history, thus eliminating the need to use CPRs to screen for fracture or ligamentous injury.[6,7]

**PT diagnosis:** Currently there are no CPRs available to diagnose patellofemoral pain syndrome; however, based on the patient's pain location, aggravating factors, special testing, and postural presentation, a diagnosis of left patellofemoral pain syndrome is appropriate.[1,5,8,9]

## Intervention

Orthotics: The decision to use orthotics in this case is unclear. The patient does not possess any of the individual predictor variables identified in the study by Sutlive et al[2]; however, she does meet three of the four variables identified in the CPR by Vicenzino et al,[4] indicating a moderate shift in probability that she will benefit from prefabricated orthotics. Given the low risk, moderate cost, and possible benefit involved in this intervention, a trial of prefabricated orthotics is indicated.

| Orthotics—Sutlive[2] | Variable Present |
|---|---|
| Forefoot valgus ≥ 2° | No |
| Great toe extension ≤ 78° | No |
| Navicular drop ≤ 3 mm | No |

| Orthotics—Vicenzino[4] | Variable Present |
|---|---|
| Age > 25 | Yes |
| Height < 165 cm | Yes |
| Worst pain < 53.25 mm on VAS | Yes |
| Mid-foot width difference > 10.96 mm | No |

Lumbar manipulation: The patient meets four of the five criteria, indicating a large and conclusive shift in probability that she will significantly improve her pain level as well as functioning if she receives lumbopelvic manipulation.[1]

| Lumbar Manipulation[1] | Variable Present |
|---|---|
| Hip IR difference > 14° | Yes |
| Ankle dorsiflexion (DF) > 16° | Yes |
| Navicular drop > 3 mm | Yes |
| No self-report of stiffness when sitting > 30 min | No |
| Squatting reported as most painful activity | Yes |

Patellar taping: The patient meets both criteria, indicating a small but perhaps important shift in the probability that she will exhibit a significant reduction in pain or an immediate improvement in functioning from patellar taping with a medial glide.[3]

| Patellar Taping[3] | Variable Present |
|---|---|
| Tibial varum > 5° | Yes |
| Positive patellar tilt test | Yes |

## Discussion

This case illustrates the clinical decision making that may be used when considering multiple Level IV interventional CPRs. In this instance it is recommended that interventions are prioritized based on the strength of the evidence. For this patient, the strongest evidence available for treatment of PFPS includes an impairment-based, regional approach to strengthening and stretching of the entire lower quarter.[10–12] In addition to the strong evidence supporting a lower-quarter impairment-based approach, the treating clinician may also consider the derivation-level CPRs.

We recommend five strategies to help improve the likelihood of success with CPR utilization. First, consider the details of the CPR in question before incorporating this into practice. Second, choose CPRs with high-quality scores, thus eliminating potential bias in their findings. Third, select a CPR that was studied in populations similar to your intended patient. Fourth, consider the strength of the +LR when prioritizing treatments, and, lastly, always test a functional or impairment-based measure before and after performing the intervention in question. This test–retest approach will provide immediate feedback concerning the effectiveness of the intervention. In the current case, the patient meets the criteria for the lumbopelvic manipulation CPR, the taping CPR, and the orthotics CPR.[1,3,4] Our patient meets all inclusion/exclusion criteria for the three CPRs, except for eligibility of military health care benefits; however, only the taping CPR has a quality score greater than 60%. Therefore, a trial of taping should be prioritized ahead of manipulation and orthotics. The lumbopelvic manipulation and orthotic CPR have low methodological-quality scores; thus if implemented, they should be used with caution. In this case the treating therapist may consider that both interventions have been studied in prior research and have found to be beneficial in individuals with patellofemoral pain syndrome.[13–15] For this reason, if it is determined that exercise and taping have not achieved their desired effects, implementation of manipulation and orthotics would be appropriate. Finally, as our patient is similar to both derivation populations, the use of lumbopelvic manipulation should be prioritized above the use of the orthotics due to its larger +LR.

This case illustrates the use of multiple derivation-level CPRs in clinical decision making. Arguments have been made that Level IV CPRs are not appropriate for use in clinical decision making. We believe that they are one component of the best current evidence that exists on a continuum of quality and generalizability. We believe that if clinicians consider Level IV CPRs in these terms as outlined above, they can be useful, along with clinical experience and patient preference, to help improve evidence-based clinical decision making.

## References

1. Iverson CA, Sutlive TG, Crowell MS, et al. Lumbopelvic manipulation for the treatment of patients with patellofemoral pain syndrome: development of a clinical prediction rule. *J Orthop Sports Phys Ther*. 2008;38:297–309.

2. Sutlive TG, Mitchell SD, Maxfield SN, et al. Identification of individuals with patellofemoral pain whose symptoms improved after a combined program of foot orthosis use and modified activity: a preliminary investigation. *Phys Ther*. 2004;84:49–61.

3. Lesher JD, Sutlive TG, Miller GA, Chine NJ, Garber MB, Wainner RS. Development of a clinical prediction rule for classifying patients with patellofemoral pain syndrome who respond to patellar taping. *J Orthop Sports Phys Ther*. 2006;36:854–866.

4. Vicenzino B, Collins N, Cleland J, McPoil T. A clinical prediction rule for identifying patients with patellofemoral pain who are likely to benefit from foot orthoses: a preliminary determination. *Br J Sports Med*. Epub ahead of print.

5. Nijs J, Van Geel C, Van der Auwera C, Van de Velde B. Diagnostic value of five clinical tests in patellofemoral pain syndrome. *Man Ther*. 2006;11:69–77.

6. Stiell IG, Greenberg GH, Wells GA, et al. Derivation of a decision rule for the use of radiography in acute knee injuries. *Ann Emerg Med*. 1995;26:405–413.

7. Seaberg DC, Jackson R. Clinical decision rule for knee radiographs. *Am J Emerg Med*. 1994;12:541–543.

8. Gerbino PG, Griffin ED, d'Hemecourt PA, et al. Patellofemoral pain syndrome: evaluation of location and intensity of pain. *Clin J Pain*. 2006;22:154–159.

9. Hamstra-Wright KL, Swanik CB, Ennis TY, Swanik KA. Joint stiffness and pain in individuals with patellofemoral syndrome. *J Orthop Sports Phys Ther*. 2005;35:495–501.

10. Reiman MP, Bolgla LA, Lorenz D. Hip functions influence on knee dysfunction: a proximal link to a distal problem. *J Sport Rehabil*. 2009;18:33–46.

11. Heintjes E, Berger MY, Bierma-Zeinstra SMA, et al. Exercise therapy for patellofemoral pain syndrome. *Cochrane Database Syst Rev*. 2003;(4):CD003472.

12. Lowry CD, Cleland JA, Dyke K. Management of patients with patellofemoral pain syndrome using a multimodal approach: a case series. *J Orthop Sports Phys Ther*. 2008;38:691–702.

13. Suter E, McMorland G, Herzog W, Bray R. Conservative lower back treatment reduces inhibition in knee-extensor muscles: a randomized controlled trial. *J Manipulative Physiol Ther*. 2000;23:76–80.

14. Suter E, McMorland G, Herzog W, Bray R. Decrease in quadriceps inhibition after sacroiliac joint manipulation in patients with anterior knee pain. *J Manipulative Physiol Ther*. 1999;22:149–153.

15. Gross MT, Foxworth JL. The role of foot orthoses as an intervention for patellofemoral pain. *J Orthop Sports Phys Ther*. 2003;33:661–670.

CASE STUDY

# Lumbar Spine

## Historical Exam

A 32-year-old male computer programmer presents to physical therapy with a 10-day history of right lower lumbar pain that does not radiate into either buttock or lower extremity. Pain occurred several hours after doing yard work that involved approximately 4 hours of heavy lifting and repetitive forward bending.

**Aggravating factors:** Forward bending, sitting greater than 15 minutes

**Relieving factors:** Rest, lying on back with knees bent, pillow under knees

**PMH:** Three episodes of mild low back pain in the past 5 years; pain usually dissipates within 2–3 days without treatment; otherwise his PMH was unremarkable

| Self-Report Outcome Measures | |
|---|---|
| Modified Oswestry Disability Index (ODI) | 34% |
| Numeric Pain Rating Scale (NPRS): Current | 4/10 |
| Numeric Pain Rating Scale (NPRS): Worst in past 24 hours | 8/10 |
| Numeric Pain Rating Scale (NPRS): Best in past 24 hours | 4/10 |
| Fear Avoidance Belief Questionnaire Work Subscale (FABQ-W) | 4 |
| Fear Avoidance Belief Questionnaire Physical Activity Subscale (FABQ-PA) | 7 |
| Modified Somatic Perception Questionnaire (MSPQ) | 5 |

## Physical Exam

**Myotomes and dermatomes:** Intact bilaterally

**Reflexes:** All 2+ bilaterally

**Posture:** Slight forward head posture with rounded shoulders; decreased kyphosis at mid-thoracic spine; increased lumbar lordosis; symmetrical height of iliac crests, ASIS, PSIS, greater trochanters, and gluteal folds

Active Range of Motion (AROM):

| Inclinometry | |
|---|---|
| Lumbar flexion | 44° to onset of comparable symptoms 7/10; no aberrant motion |
| Lumbar extension | 22° with mild increase in symptoms 5/10 |
| Lumbar right side bending | 20° with mild increase in symptoms 5/10 |
| Lumbar left side bending | 12° with comparable symptoms 6–7/10 |
| Hip internal rotation | 40° bilaterally without a change in symptoms |
| Straight leg raise | 50–60° bilaterally without a change in symptoms |

**Passive intervertebral motion:** P-A spring testing; hypomobile throughout the thoracic and lumbar spine with reproduction of comparable symptoms at L4 and L5 with central and right-sided P-A springing; no hypermobility noted in the lumbar spine

## Special Tests

**Slump and SLR:** Negative for adverse neural tension bilaterally

**Repeated flexion/repeated extension:** No effect on location of symptoms

**Sacroiliac (SI) testing (Gaenslen's, femoral shear, SI compression, SI distraction, sacral provocation):** Negative for pain reproduction

**Prone instability test:** Negative for pain reduction

# Clinical Decision Making

## Diagnosis/Classification

Research has indicated the diagnostic and prognostic shortcomings of a pathoanatomical approach to low back pain.[1,2] Despite this fact, identifying the area of the patient's primary complaint may be beneficial in directing treatment. For this reason, the CPR that pertains to the pathoanatomical diagnosis of pain arising from the sacroiliac joint was used. However, this diagnosis is unlikely given that the patient does not possess any of the predictor variables identified by Laslett et al.[3] as predictive of sacroiliac pain, indicating a large and conclusive shift that the condition is absent.

| Diagnosis of SI Pain[3] | Variable Present |
|---|---|
| SI compression | No |
| SI distraction | No |
| Femoral shear | No |
| Sacral provocation | No |
| Gaenslen's right | No |
| Gaenslen's left | No |

## Prognosis

Hancock et al.[4] have derived a prediction rule to identify patients with LBP who will rapidly recover regardless of treatment received. This patient does not meet any of the three identified criteria, thus eliminating our ability to predict prognosis based on these interventions.

| Recovery from LBP[4] | Variable Present |
|---|---|
| Baseline pain ≤ 7/10 | No |
| Duration of current episode ≤ 5 days | No |
| Number of previous episodes ≤ 1 | No |

## PT Classification/Treatment

Lumbopelvic manipulation: The use of a treatment-based classification system as originally described by Delitto et al.[5] has demonstrated improved outcomes in the PT management of low back pain.[6,7] Primary subgroups include "manipulation," "stabilization," and "specific exercise," with a currently emerging "traction" classification. According to this treatment-based classification system, this patient is best classified as "manipulation." He meets 5/5 criteria, indicating a large and conclusive shift in the probability that he will likely have a 50% improvement in LBP-related disability from lumbopelvic manipulation and exercise.[8]

| Lumbar Manipulation[8] | Variable Present |
|---|---|
| Pain does not travel below the knee | Yes |
| Onset ≤ 16 days ago | Yes |
| Lumbar hypomobility (via P-A mobs) | Yes |
| One hip has > 35° of internal rotation | Yes |
| FABQ- Work subscale score ≤ 19 | Yes |

Lumbar stabilization: The patient does not fit well into the stabilization subgroup as he meets only one of the four predictor variables indicating that he would benefit from lumbar stabilization.[9] Additionally, he meets all four variables from a CPR indicating likely failure with a stabilization approach.

| Failure with Stabilization[9] | Variable Present |
|---|---|
| FABQ—Physical Activity < 8 | Yes |
| Aberrant movement absent | Yes |
| No hypermobility during P-A spring | Yes |
| Negative prone instability | Yes |

Specific exercise: Currently a CPR does not exist to identify patients who will benefit from "specific exercise direction"; however, given that his symptoms do not radiate from the low back and no directional preference was elicited in the examination, it would not be likely he will benefit from specific exercise.[10]

Traction: This patient also meets all four criteria of a CPR for lumbar traction in a supine position, indicating a moderate shift in probability that he will benefit from this treatment.[11]

| Supine Traction[11] | Variable Present |
|---|---|
| FABQ—Work subscale < 21 | Yes |
| No neurological deficits | Yes |
| Age > 30 | Yes |
| Nonmanual work job status | Yes |

Facet joint injections: As part of the differential diagnosis process it is the responsibility of the examining therapist to consider treatment options beyond those described within the PT scope of practice. For this reason the CPR identifying patients with low back pain who may or may not respond well to facet block injection is considered. This patient only met two of the seven criteria, indicating a large and conclusive shift in probability that he is not likely to benefit from this type of treatment.[12]

| Facet Block[12] | Variable Present |
| --- | --- |
| Age ≥ 50 | No |
| Symptoms best with walking | No |
| Symptoms best with sitting | No |
| Onset pain is paraspinal | Yes |
| Positive extension rotation test | No |
| Modified Somatic Perception Questionnaire (MSPQ) > 13 | No |
| Absence of centralization | Yes |

## Discussion

This case illustrates the use of CPRs in a patient with low back pain to help rule out possible pathoanatomical medical diagnoses, determine whether the patient's symptoms are likely to improve without treatment, and to guide physical therapy treatment. As with the cervicothoracic region and knee cases, many of the CPRs utilized are Level IV, thus necessitating careful consideration of both the quality of the study as well as the specifics of the study (e.g., patient characteristics, inclusion/exclusion criteria, LR size) to determine whether the findings are applicable to the patient.

A diagnosis of pain arising from the sacroiliac joint is unlikely due to the location of symptoms (lower back only), as well as the cluster of tests by Laslett et al.[3] However, it is important to highlight that the methodology of this study is different than a true CPR, and currently an assessment tool to evaluate the quality of Level IV diagnostic CPRs has not been established. For this reason caution should be exercised when using this rule despite the similarity between our patient and the study's sample.

Prognosis for this patient cannot be established using the Hancock et al. CPR, as the patient does not meet any of the three predictor variables identified.[4] However, given that the patient is young and healthy with a past history of infrequent LBP of short duration, recovery from this episode of LBP is likely with PT intervention.

Treatment-based classification through the use of the above CPRs indicates that the patient best fits into the "manipulation" subgroup, as he meets five of five criteria for the validated manipulation CPR. In this case, the patient is similar to the populations of both the derivation and validation studies so the CPR may be used with confidence.[8,13] Prognosis for success with PT is influenced as the patient meets all the criteria for the CPR, indicating a large and conclusive shift in probability that he will experience a greater than 50% reduction in disability after only two sessions of manipulation and exercise as well as significant decreases in medication use, continued medical treatment, or time missed from work due to LBP at 6 months.[13] Given the similarity of our subject and the study populations along with the favorable prognosis for this patient after manipulation, this technique is strongly recommended in this case.

Other possible subgroups that may be considered for this patient are "stabilization" or "traction." In this case, a comprehensive lumbar stabilization program is unlikely to provide adequate relief as the patient has met all four criteria indicating failure with specific stabilization.[9]

There are two CPRs available to identify patients who may benefit from traction. One found that subjects with either peripheralization with repeated extension or a crossed SLR had greater short-term benefit from prone traction.[14] However, our patient does not meet the inclusion criteria of this study, as his symptoms did not change with repeated movements, and his crossed SLR was negative.

The second traction CPR identifies patients likely to benefit from traction performed in the supine position.[11] Our patient is similar to the subjects in this derivation study, and the quality score of the study was 78%, which is above the recommended 60%.[15,16] Therefore, given the low risk and possible benefit (50% reduction in disability within three sessions) from supine traction, this treatment may be worth including. Due to the Level IV status of the supine traction CPR, it is advisable to retest the patient after the intervention to ensure progress. An example of this would be retesting in the standing forward bending position with an inclinometer to determine whether the AROM before symptom onset has improved.

This case study demonstrates the preferential weighting of a validated CPR over a Level IV CPR in clinical decision making within the framework of a treatment-based classification system. These CPRs allow the clinician to confidently migrate toward the treatment threshold and subsequently use the response to the initial treatment as an additional finding to help guide the ongoing clinical decision-making process. It is worth highlighting once again that CPRs should never be used in isolation rather than as a component of the best available evidence in conjunction with patient values and clinical experience.

## References

1. Abenhaim L, Rossignol M, Gobeille D, Bonvalot Y, Fines P, Scott S. The prognostic consequences in the making of the initial medical diagnosis of work-related back injuries. *Spine.* 1995:791–795.

2. Kleinstück F, Dvorak J. Mannion AF. Are "structural abnormalities" on magnetic resonance imaging a contraindication to the successful conservative treatment of chronic nonspecific low back pain? *Spine.* 2006;31:2250–2257.

3. Laslett M, Aprill CN, McDonald B, Yourn SB. Diagnosis of sacroiliac joint pain: validity of individual provocation tests and composites of tests. *Man Ther.* 2005;10:207–218.

4. Hancock MJ, Maher CG, Latimer J, Herbert RD, McAuley JH. Can rate of recovery be predicted in patients with acute low back pain? Development of a clinical prediction rule. *Eur J Pain.* 2009;13:51–55.

5. Delitto A, Erhard RE, Bowling RW. A treatment-based classification approach to low back syndrome: identifying and staging patients for conservative treatment. *Phys Ther.* 1995;75:470–489.

6. Brennan GP, Fritz JM, Hunter SJ, Thackeray A, Delitto A, Erhard RE. Identifying subgroups of patients with acute/subacute "nonspecific" low back pain: results of a randomized clinical trial. *Spine.* 2006;31:623–631.

7. Fritz JM, Cleland JA, Childs JD. Subgrouping patients with low back pain: evolution of a classification approach to physical therapy. *J Orthop Sports Phys Ther.* 2007;37:290–302.

8. Flynn T, Fritz J, Whitman J, et al. A clinical prediction rule for classifying patients with low back pain who demonstrate short-term improvement with spinal manipulation. *Spine.* 2002;27:2835–2843.

9. Hicks GE, Fritz JM, Delitto A, McGill SM. Preliminary development of a clinical prediction rule for determining which patients with low back pain will respond to a stabilization exercise program. *Arch Phys Med Rehabil.* 2005;86:1753–1762.

10. Long A, Donelson R, Fung T. Does it matter which exercise? A randomized control trial of exercise for low back pain. *Spine.* 2004;29:2593–2602.

11. Cai C, Pua Y, Lim K. A clinical prediction rule for classifying patients with low back pain who demonstrate short-term improvement with mechanical lumbar traction. *Eur Spine J.* 2009;18:554–561.

12. Laslett M, McDonald B, Aprill CN, Tropp H, Oberg B. Clinical predictors of screening lumbar zygapophyseal joint blocks: development of clinical prediction rules. *Spine J.* 6:370–379.

13. Childs JD, Fritz JM, Flynn TW, et al. A clinical prediction rule to identify patients with low back pain most likely to benefit from spinal manipulation: a validation study. *Ann Intern Med.* 2004;141:920–928.

14. Fritz JM, Lindsay W, Matheson JW, et al. Is there a subgroup of patients with low back pain likely to benefit from mechanical traction? Results of a randomized clinical trial and subgrouping analysis. *Spine.* 2007;32:E793–E800.

15. Beneciuk JM, Bishop MD, George SZ. Clinical prediction rules for physical therapy interventions: a systematic review. *Phys Ther.* 2009;89:114–124.

16. Kuijpers T, van der Windt DAWM, van der Heijden GJMG, Bouter LM. Systematic review of prognostic cohort studies on shoulder disorders. *Pain.* 2004;109:420–431.

## CASE STUDY

# Foot/Ankle

## Historical Exam

A 23-year-old recreational basketball player with a history of recurrent ankle sprains presents to physical therapy after injuring his right ankle 2 days ago while playing basketball. He describes landing on another player's foot with a subsequent inversion and plantarflexion injury. He was able to bear weight with significant pain and limping immediately after the injury. He also notes significant swelling and lateral pain during all weight-bearing activities. He has been using rest, ice, compression, elevation, and crutches over the past 2 days.

**Aggravating factors:** Any right LE weight-bearing activities; symptoms are worse in the evening

**Relieving factors:** Rest, ice, ibuprofen

**PMH:** Recurrent bilateral ankle sprains

| Self-Report Items | |
|---|---|
| Lower Extremity Functional Scale (LEFS) | 36/80 |
| Numeric Pain Rating Scale (NPRS): Current | 3/10 ache at rest |
| Numeric Pain Rating Scale (NPRS): Worst in past 24 hours | 7/10 sharp lateral ankle with weight bearing |
| Numeric Pain Rating Scale (NPRS): Best in past 24 hours | 3/10 ache |

## Physical Exam

**Observation:** Right lateral ankle swelling with ecchymosis over the lateral malleolus down to the lateral mid-foot; right foot/ankle resting position of plantarflexion

**Gait:** Significantly antalgic on the right with absence of heel strike; onset of 7/10 pain immediately upon weight bearing, but he is able to tolerate walking 20 feet

**Palpation:** Tenderness to palpation of the right sinus tarsi and the right tip and inferior/posterior margin of fibula; no tenderness in metatarsals, base of the fifth metatarsal, cuboid, or medial structures

ROM:

| Ankle Inversion (Goniometer) | Right | Left |
|---|---|---|
| AROM—Sitting | 40° | 18° with pain |
| PROM—Sitting | 42° | 18° with pain |

| Ankle Eversion (Goniometer) | Right | Left |
|---|---|---|
| AROM—Sitting | 20° | 6° with pain |
| PROM—Sitting | 22° | 7° with pain |

| Ankle Plantarflexion (Goniometer) | Right | Left |
|---|---|---|
| AROM—Supine | 48° | 32° with pain |
| PROM—Supine | 50° | 33° with pain |

| Ankle Dorsiflexion (Goniometer) | Right | Left |
|---|---|---|
| AROM—Prone knee extended | 7° | −15° with pain |
| PROM—Prone knee extended | 8° | −15° with pain |
| AROM—Prone knee flexed | 10° | −15° with pain |
| PROM—Prone knee flexed | 14° | −15° with pain |

**Joint mobility:** Unable to examine due to pain and swelling

**Special tests:** Anterior drawer, talar tilt, navicular drop; unable to examine due to pain and swelling

**Figure 8 (cm):** 56.3 on the right; 54.1 on the left

**Manual muscle test:** Not examined due to pain

## Clinical Decision Making

### Diagnosis

**Appropriateness for PT:** Possible foot or ankle fracture; based on the history and physical examination, radiographs are not needed to rule out a mid-foot fracture as the patient does not meet any of the four criteria of the Ottawa Foot Rules.[1]

| Ottawa Foot Rules[1] | Variable Present |
|---|---|
| Inability to bear weight immediately after injury | No |
| Inability to bear weight during examination | No |
| Tenderness at base of fifth metatarsal | No |
| Tenderness at the navicular | No |

However, this patient does have tenderness at the tip and posterior edge of the lateral malleolus, and a fracture cannot be ruled out with confidence using the Ottawa Ankle Rules.[1] Given the risk of delaying medical treatment for a possible fracture the patient should be referred to a physician for examination and radiographs to rule out ankle fracture before initiation or continuation of PT.

| Ottawa Ankle Rules[1] | Variable Present |
|---|---|
| Inability to bear weight immediately after injury | No |
| Inability to bear weight during examination | No |
| Tenderness at tip or distal 6 cm of medial malleolus | No |
| Tenderness at tip or distal 6 cm of lateral malleolus | Yes |

## Discussion

In this case, a Level I CPR was used to determine the appropriateness of initiating PT. Even in validated CPRs it is important to consider how similar our subject is to those used to derive or validate the CPR. In this case, our subject is similar in age, acuity, and activity level of the subjects in the derivation and several validation studies.[2–5] Additionally, although this CPR was derived using ED physicians performing the tests, it has also been validated for use by PTs.[5] The application of this CPR to our patient is appropriate and since ankle fracture cannot be ruled out, referral to a physician for examination is necessary prior to continuing with PT treatment.

This case highlights the use of a Level I screening CPR to help determine the appropriateness of continuing PT in a direct access situation. The patient did not meet all of the criteria necessary to confidently rule out an ankle fracture and therefore the patient should be referred for radiograph prior to continuing PT.

### References

1. Stiell IG, Greenberg GH, McKnight RD, et al. A study to develop clinical decision rules for the use of radiography in acute ankle injuries. *Ann Emerg Med.* 1992;21:384–390.
2. Stiell IG, Greenberg GH, McKnight RD, et al. Decision rules for the use of radiography in acute ankle injuries. Refinement and prospective validation. *JAMA.* 1993;269:1127–1132.

3.  Pigman EC, Klug RK, Sanford S, Jolly BT. Evaluation of the Ottawa clinical decision rules for the use of radiography in acute ankle and midfoot injuries in the emergency department: an independent site assessment. *Ann Emerg Med*. 1994;24:41–45.

4.  Leddy JJ, Smolinski RJ, Lawrence J, Snyder JL, Priore RL. Prospective evaluation of the Ottawa Ankle Rules in a university sports medicine center. With a modification to increase specificity for identifying malleolar fractures. *Am J Sports Med*. 1998;26:158–165.

5.  Springer BA, Arciero RA, Tenuta JJ, Taylor DC. A prospective study of modified Ottawa ankle rules in a military population. *Am J Sports Med*. 2000;28:864–868.

# CPR Quality Scores of Level IV Prognostic Studies

| Question<br>Study | A | B | C | D | E | F | G | H | I | J | K | L | M | N | O | P | Q | R | Total |
|---|---|---|---|---|---|---|---|---|---|---|---|---|---|---|---|---|---|---|---|
| *Cervical Spine* | | | | | | | | | | | | | | | | | | | |
| Cleland et al. 2007<br>(see page 101) | No | No | Yes | Yes | Yes | Yes | No | Yes | Yes | No | Yes | Yes | No | Yes | Yes | Yes | Yes | No | 72% |
| Hartling et al. 2002<br>(see page 99) | No | No | Yes | Yes | No | Yes | Yes | Yes | No | No | Yes | No | Yes | Yes | Yes | Yes | Yes | No | 61% |

# CPR Quality Scores of Level IV Intervention Studies

| Question Study | A | B | C | D | E | F | G | H | I | J | K | L | M | N | O | P | Q | R | Total |
|---|---|---|---|---|---|---|---|---|---|---|---|---|---|---|---|---|---|---|---|
| **Cervical Spine** | | | | | | | | | | | | | | | | | | | |
| Cleland et al. 2007 (see page 108) | No | No | Yes | Yes | Yes | No | Yes | No | Yes | Yes | No | Yes | Yes | Yes | Yes | Yes | Yes | No | 67% |
| Emshoff et al. 2008 (see page 118) | No | Yes | Yes | Yes | Yes | Yes | No | No | Yes | Yes | No | Yes | No | Yes | Yes | Yes | Yes | Yes | 72% |
| Fernandez-de-las-Penas et al. 2008 (see page 110) | No | No | Yes | Yes | Yes | No | Yes | Yes | No | Yes | No | Yes | Yes | Yes | Yes | Yes | Yes | No | 67% |
| Raney et al. 2009 (see page 115) | No | No | Yes | Yes | Yes | No | Yes | No | Yes | Yes | No | Yes | Yes | Yes | Yes | Yes | Yes | No | 67% |
| Tseng et al. 2006 (see page 104) | No | No | Yes | No | No | No | Yes | Yes | Yes | Yes | Yes | Yes | No | Yes | Yes | Yes | Yes | No | 61% |
| **Lumbar Spine** | | | | | | | | | | | | | | | | | | | |
| Alonso-Blanco et al. 2009 (see page 177) | No | Yes | Yes | No | Yes | No | Yes | Yes | Yes | Yes | No | Yes | Yes | Yes | Yes | Yes | Yes | No | 72% |
| Cai et al. 2009 (see page 173) | No | No | Yes | Yes | Yes | No | Yes | Yes | Yes | Yes | No | Yes | Yes | Yes | Yes | Yes | Yes | No | 72% |
| Hicks et al. 2005 *Failure* (see page 159) | No | No | Yes | Yes | Yes | No | Yes | No | Yes | Yes | No | Yes | Yes | Yes | Yes | Yes | Yes | No | 67% |
| Hicks et al. 2005 *Success* (see page 159) | No | No | Yes | Yes | Yes | No | Yes | No | Yes | Yes | No | Yes | Yes | Yes | Yes | Yes | Yes | Yes | 72% |
| Fritz et al. 2004 (see page 167) | No | No | Yes | Yes | Yes | No | Yes | No | Yes | Yes | No | Yes | Yes | Yes | Yes | Yes | No | No | 61% |
| Fritz et al. 2007 (see page 171) | No | No | Yes | Yes | Yes | No | Yes | Yes | No | Yes | Yes | Yes | No | Yes | Yes | Yes | No | No | 61% |
| Laslett et al. 2006 (see page 175) | No | No | Yes | No | No | No | Yes | Yes | No | Yes | Yes | Yes | Yes | Yes | No | Yes | Yes | No | 56% |

| | 1 | 2 | 3 | 4 | 5 | 6 | 7 | 8 | 9 | 10 | 11 | 12 | 13 | 14 | 15 | 16 | 17 | 18 | |
|---|---|---|---|---|---|---|---|---|---|---|---|---|---|---|---|---|---|---|---|
| **Shoulder** | | | | | | | | | | | | | | | | | | | |
| Mintken et al. 2009 (see page 144) | No | No | Yes | Yes | Yes | No | Yes | Yes | Yes | Yes | No | Yes | Yes | Yes | Yes | Yes | Yes | No | 72% |
| **Elbow** | | | | | | | | | | | | | | | | | | | |
| Vicenzino et al. 2009 (see page 137) | No | Yes | No | Yes | Yes | No | Yes | No | No | Yes | Yes | Yes | No | Yes | Yes | Yes | Yes | Yes | 67% |
| **Knee** | | | | | | | | | | | | | | | | | | | |
| Currier et al. 2007 (see page 208) | No | No | No | Yes | Yes | No | Yes | Yes | Yes | Yes | No | Yes | No | Yes | Yes | No | Yes | No | 56% |
| Iverson et al. 2008 (see page 195) | No | No | Yes | Yes | No | No | Yes | No | Yes | Yes | No | Yes | No | Yes | Yes | Yes | Yes | No | 56% |
| Lesher et al. 2006 (see page 198) | No | No | Yes | Yes | No | No | Yes | Yes | Yes | Yes | No | Yes | No | Yes | Yes | Yes | Yes | Yes | 67% |
| Sutlive et al. 2004 (see page 203) | No | No | Yes | Yes | Yes | No | Yes | No | Yes | Yes | No | Yes | No | Yes | Yes | Yes | Yes | No | 61% |
| Vicenzino et al. 2009 (see page 200) | No | Yes | No | Yes | Yes | No | No | No | No | Yes | No | Yes | No | Yes | Yes | Yes | Yes | No | 50% |
| **Ankle** | | | | | | | | | | | | | | | | | | | |
| Whitman et al. 2009 (see page 214) | No | Yes | Yes | Yes | Yes | No | Yes | Yes | Yes | Yes | No | Yes | Yes | Yes | Yes | Yes | Yes | Yes | 83% |

# Quality Assessment of Diagnostic CPRs

| Item | Description | Yes | No |
|---|---|---|---|
| 1. | Inception cohort | | |
| 2. | Prospective and consecutive subjective enrollment | | |
| 3. | Description of setting | | |
| 4. | Description of subject's baseline demographics | | |
| 5. | Clear inclusion/exclusion criteria | | |
| 6. | Recognized valid/reliable reference standard | | |
| 7. | Explanation for predictor variable selection | | |
| 8. | Reliable predictor variables (ICC $\geq$ 0.70; Kappa $\geq$ 0.60) | | |
| 9. | Prospective application of reference standard within a reasonable time frame after the examination | | |
| 10. | Detailed description of positive/negative on reference standard | | |
| 11. | Blinded examiner | | |
| 12. | Blinded interpretation of reference standard | | |
| 13. | Diagnostic accuracy of significant individual predictor variables reported | | |
| 14. | Variables exceeding set cut score for univariate significance entered into regression model | | |
| 15. | Results of regression analysis reported with 95% CIs | | |
| 16. | Statistical significance of the model reported | | |
| 17. | Full description of retained predictor variables presented | | |
| 18. | Ten to 15 subjects per variable presented in the final clinical prediction rule | | |
| 19. | Were study withdrawals/dropouts < 10% | | |
| | **Total** | | |

# CPR Quality Scores of Interventional Validation Studies

| Question Study | 10 | 11 | 12 | 13 | 14 | 15 | 16 | 17 | 18 | 19 | Total |
|---|---|---|---|---|---|---|---|---|---|---|---|
| **Lumbar Spine** | | | | | | | | | | | |
| Childs et al. 2004 (see page 163) | 1 | 1 | 1 | 1 | 1 | 0 | 0 | 0 | 0 | 0 | 50% |
| Hancock et al. 2008 (see page 163) | 1 | 1 | 1 | 1 | 0 | 1 | 0 | 0 | 0 | 0 | 50% |
| **Shoulder** | | | | | | | | | | | |
| Kuijpers et al. 2007 (see page 132) | 1 | 1 | 1 | 1 | 0 | 0 | 0 | 0 | 0 | 0 | 40% |

# CPR Decision-Making Algorithm

*Is it appropriate for me to apply the results to my patient's treatment?*

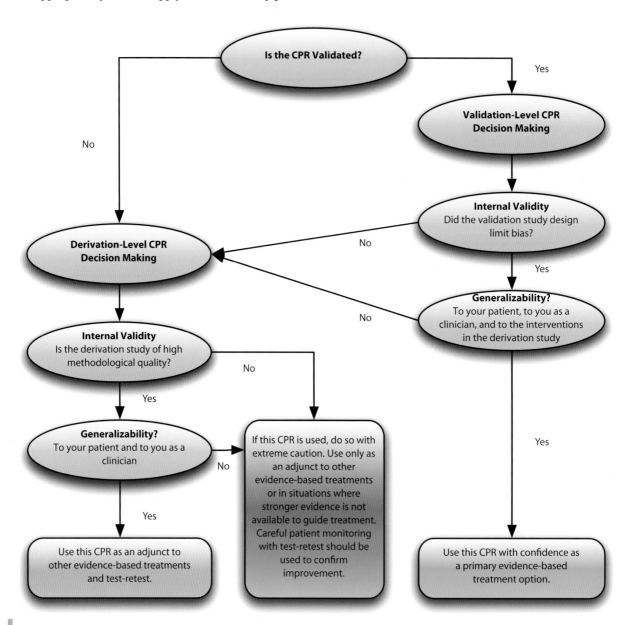

Health Sciences Library
University of Saskatchewan Libraries
Room B205 Health Sciences Building
107 WIGGINS ROAD
SASKATOON, SK  S7N 5E5  CANADA

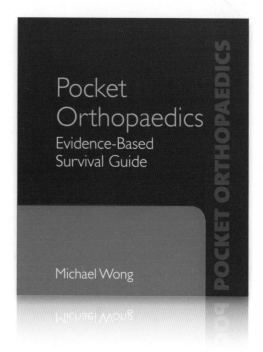

**Also Available: From Michael Wong**

Pocket Orthopaedics:
Evidence-Based Survival Guide

Michael Wong, DPT, OCS, FAAOMPT
Associate Professor, Azusa Pacific University
Staff Therapist, Outpatient Rehabilitation,
 Loma Linda University Medical Center
Staff Therapist, Corina Hills Sports Medicine

ISBN-13: 978-0-7637-5075-6
Spiral/paperback ■ 408 Pages ■ © 2011

*Pocket Orthopaedics: Evidence-Based Survival Guide* is a comprehensive resource for students in any orthopaedic course and is designed for physicians, physical therapists and assistants, chiropractors, athletic trainers, and other health professionals. The handbook's user-friendly format enables readers to locate information quickly and easily. Organized by body region, chapters include red flags for potentially serious conditions, information on key tests and outcomes, and algorithms for diagnosis. Also included are medical screening differential diagnosis tables, origin, insertion, nerve supply, and action of muscles. The text includes useful suggestions and considerations for evaluation, post-surgical rehabilitation protocols, and evidence-based parameters for modalities. Durable and pocket-sized, yet comprehensive, this quick reference is an exceptional learning tool for students and those already working in the field.

**Features**

- ■ Convenient access to key topics
- ■ Important information and resources for accurate diagnosis and treatment
- ■ A straightforward approach to high-quality care
- ■ Hundreds of color photos and illustrations

**Order Your Copy Today!**

Visit www.jbpub.com/healthprofessions or call 1-800-832-0034.